SPORT SPECIFIC AEROBIC ROUTINES

by

Dr. Leon Greene
Associate Professor and Program Coordinator
HPER Department
University of Kansas
Lawrence, Kansas

eddie bowers publishing company
2600 JACKSON STREET
DUBUQUE, IA 52001

The Author

Dr. Leon Greene is Associate Professor and Program Coordinator, Health, Physical Education and Recreation Department, University of Kansas. There he coached basketball, tennis, snow skiing, and cross country; he also directed the Elementary Physical Education Laboratory at the University of Kansas for 14 years. He co-directed the KU Sports Skills and Fitness School for Children for 7 years, and has been an active member in AAPHERD for 17 years.

Acknowledgments

I am very grateful to several individuals who helped me on this book. I extend a special thanks to the Childrens' Dance and Aerobic Rhythms Class of 1985 who helped develop the concept of Sport Aerobics. I especially thank Renee Powell, Mary Allen, and Mickey Greene for serving as models in the photographs and for taking the time to demonstrate their skills. I appreciate Marsha Duff's review of chapters two and four and her comments relative to choreography. Finally, I thank the many teachers who shared their knowledge and expertise with me.

eddie bowers publishing company
2600 JACKSON STREET
DUBUQUE, IA 52001

ISBN 0-912855-91-6

Table of Contents

Table of Contents
(continued)

Table of Figures

PREFACE

In general, people will not exercise if they do not enjoy it. Although the nation seems to be in a physical fitness boom, the percentage of people exercising on a regular basis is still low compared to what might be expected as the result of a trend. The question remains, among the physical education, health and other related professions, as to whether or not contemporary physical fitness activities are really designed for participation by a large percentage of the population.

The purpose of this book is to provide a new and somewhat different approach to aerobic rhythms and dance. This approach makes use of sport related skills choreographed to music. Sport activities are popular with elementary school, high school, and college students. Leisure time sport programs are also rising in popularity among all age levels of society. Sport specific aerobic routines may be the answer to aerobic exercise. More important is the fact that such routines are for individuals of all age and ability levels.

The book is divided into five parts. The material in Part One (Chapters 1-2) pertains to general information relative to research on aerobic exercise, sport skills, rhythm movement, and the benefits of sport aerobics. The information in these chapters establishes a foundation for sport specific aerobic activity and provides direction for the remaining parts of the book.

Part Two (Chapters 3-4) provide the reader with information and directions on how to choreograph sport skills to music. Once a sport specific aerobic routine is developed, it is necessary to change or modify it at various times. As an individual learns a routine, new and challenging movements help polish the sport skills and increase the fitness level. It is critical for the reader to understand how to select sport skills for a given piece of music. These chapters make this task easy.

Part Three (Chapters 5-9) lists and describes sport specific aerobic routines for sports like: basketball, volleyball, soccer, softball, and touch football. All of the routines have suggested music and are described in detail as to the movements required.

Part Four (Chapters 10-11) lists and describes sport aerobic routines for two individual sports such as tennis and track and field. These routines have suggested music and the movements required are described in detail.

Part Five (Chapters 12-13) provides the reader with information on techniques used to assess the effects of sport specific aerobic routines and/or other aerobic activity. Material is also provided on how to evaluate a routine to determine if it is choreographed appropriately and is fitness related.

At the end of some chapters, where appropriate, suggested activities to enhance the learning experience are provided for the reader. These suggestions are merely ways to practice skills and techniques for developing and practicing sport specific aerobic routines.

Illustrations and diagrams are shown throughout the text for the purpose of better explaining a given point or idea. The pictures are to give the reader a visual description of various movements and more meaning to a given routine.

References are listed at the end of each chapter. Since sport specific aerobics is a rather new concept, literature was not abundant. This is no way detracts or limits the usefulness and importance of sport specific aerobics. It is a practical approach to developing or refining sport skills and maintaining or improving fitness levels.

CHAPTER 1

SPORTS, FITNESS AND AEROBICS

In the last 15 years many changes have occurred in activities and exercises related to fitness. Running, jogging, weight programs, aerobic dance and rhythms, as well as other fitness related activities have attracted many participants. Aerobic dance and rhythms have become a vital part of the lifestyle for millions of Americans. At the same time, there are millions of Americans that are not participating in aerobic dance and rhythms, but in other forms of exercise.

Aerobic dance and rhythmical routines have been popular with certain segments of the American population. Generally, participants in this type of activity have been women. As a result, many males within the population have come to believe it is an activity for females. Most of the aerobic dance and rhythmical routines currently used contain a lot of dance oriented steps. Because of the dance step emphasis, many people find it difficult to learn routines and get a proper aerobic workout. Consequently, many people seem to be looking for alternative ways to get aerobic exercise.

SPORT ACTIVITY

Sport programs and activities are such an important part of American society that little explanation is needed as to why sport skills were selected for this type of exercise. America's youth and adults seem to spend a lot of time participating in sport related activities. It may be for fun, socialization, use of leisure time, or just a good means to release energy and get an exercise workout. Many people probably participate in sports for the exercise. What many individuals fail to realize is that they must not only have the necessary skills to participate at a given level, but also maintain a level of physical fitness that is appropriate for the sport.

Skill Execution

Sport programs in America are for all people. Included are: the skilled and the unskilled, the handicapped and the nonhandicapped, as well as the young and the old. Since sport programs seem to involve such a broad cross section of society, selecting sport skills to choreograph to music for exercise routines seemed to be appropriate. Why not develop or refine the sport skills and at the same time improve the physical fitness level? Physical fitness that relates to skills is also a partner to level of performance. The underlying concept to this would be "practice the way in which the game is to be played."

Sport Specific

Any sport activity requires specific movements for participation. The skills may range from running and jumping to dribbling and shooting a basketball. Each skill remains specific to a given sport. Skill execution requires a certain amount of energy that evolves from one's physical fitness level.

RELATIONSHIP OF RHYTHM AND FITNESS TO SKILL EXECUTION

All movement has a rhythmical component. The execution of sport skills requires movement, therefore rhythm becomes a force that may dictate the quality of the performance. Rhythm is a regular pattern of movement and/or sound. It can be felt, seen, and/or heard. All sport skills are complex movement patterns that require an individual to have skill related fitness qualities. Rhythmical movement seems to be a natural for developing and maintaining sport related skills. The important role that rhythm plays in the use of sport skills can easily be demonstrated (Figure 1.1).

[SPORT SKILLS + RHYTHM + FITNESS = QUALITY PERFORMANCE]

FIGURE 1.1. Relationship of rhythm to sport skills.

The quality will motivate and reinforce one's needs and desires to continue exercising through the medium of sport activities.

Sport Skills and Rhythm

It seems to be appropriate to add a new phase to the already exciting aerobic dance and rhythmical routines used for exercise. If various sport related skills are analyzed, it is easy to recognize the following:

1. The execution of these skills requires good rhythm.

2. Most of the skills are performed when an individual is moving (running, jogging, jumping, sprinting, etc.).

3. Each sport requires a specific type of physical fitness for the proper execution of the required skills.

4. Aerobic endurance is necessary for quality execution of the skills, therefore, possibly increasing the chance for personal enjoyment.

5. These skills require many of the same movements that are dance related at a basic level.

4

Rhythm may be the quality associated with skills that really promotes the fun and enjoyment aspect of participating in sports.

The rhythm factor makes it obvious that aerobic exercise routines to music can be developed by using sport skills as the movement. These routines may be a somewhat futuristic solution to getting more Americans participating in aerobic dance related fitness programs. In sport specific aerobic routines, there is something for everybody.

FITNESS AND SPORT SKILLS

Physical fitness seems to mean different things to different people. Regardless of how it is interpreted, most people would agree that it does enhance one's functional capacity for a better lifestyle. A better lifestyle can lead to a positive feeling and more enthusiasm for life without experiencing fatigue. A high level of physical fitness can allow for participation in activities for personal enjoyment. Many Americans participate in sport activities for this very reason.

Health and Performance

To some extent, physical fitness is two sided. There is physical fitness for motor performance and physical fitness that is more health related. A critical factor here, is that for an individual to participate in sport activities he/she must achieve a level of fitness that is both health related and motor related. This can easily be described by comparing the components of the different types of fitness as listed in Figure 1.2.

Skill Related	Health Related
Agility	Strength
Balance	Endurance
Coordination	Aerobic Fitness
Speed	Flexibility
Power	Body Composition
Reaction Time	

FIGURE 1.2. Fitness components related to skill development and health.

Although there may not be a direct relationship between these two attributes, there is certainly an indirect one.

Sport specific routines are designed to focus primarily on health related fitness. This type of exercise is unique in that there is carry over value to skill related fitness and to the improvement of sport skills. It is not often that an individual can exercise and receive health related benefits and promote leisure time sport skills at the same time. These routines are an excellent means for maximizing time needed to exercise and practice sport skills.

Movement and Fitness

There is one other relationship between fitness and sport skills. Simply, that together, because both require movement, they may help prevent individuals from encountering hypokinetic diseases. Some of these diseases that can be prevented through movement are: low back problems, coronary heart disease, overweight problems and/or obesity. Regular participation (3-4 times per week) in sport specific aerobic exercise routines, should help one greatly reduce his/her chances to deal with this type of disease.

SUMMARY

The interrelationships among sport skills, physical fitness and performance are so close, it is near impossible to remove one without drastically affecting the other two (Figure 1.3).

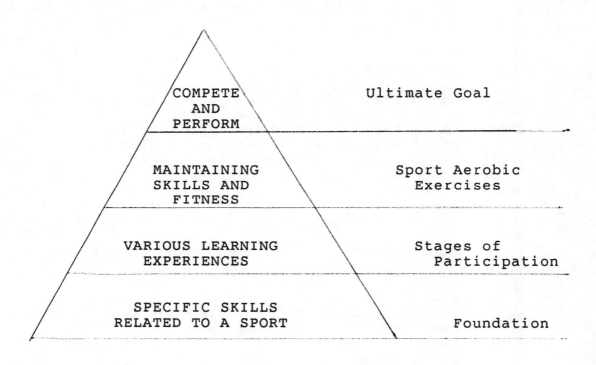

FIGURE 1.3. Interrelationship of sport skills, physical fitness, and performance.

This suggests that most individuals establish a foundation for sport participation at some point in time by acquiring some of the necessary skills and then gradually progress through various learning experiences by participating in a given sport activity. The more one participates, the more steps that individual will pass through toward the ultimate goal of competing or performing at the highest possible level. Most individuals seem to experience problems with the maintenance of the skills and fitness levels. Consequently, many people participate in sport games or activities in a somewhat unsafe manner and in a less than healthy state of being.

6

SUGGESTED ACTIVITIES

1. Select a sport skill that you can execute. Practice doing the skill several times. Try to execute the skill in slow motion and count a beat for each sequence of the movement. Repeat two to three times to make sure the number of beats is correct for the sequence. This is the beginning of being more aware of the rhythmical nature of sport skill execution.

2. After completing exercise number one, proceed to executing the skill or practicing the skill while moving as if in the actual contest. Analyze the complete movement pattern and determine what kind of rhythmical sequence you are feeling with this type of movement. By this time, you have just completed the initial phase of understanding more about sport aerobic routines.

SELECTED BIBLIOGRAPHY

Dauer, V. and Pangrazi, R. Dynamic Physical Education for Elementary School Children. 8th Ed. Edina, MN.: Burgess Publishing, 1986.

Harris, J., Pittman, A. and Waller, M. Dance A While. Minneapolis, MN: Burgess Publishing Company, 1978.

Petray, C. and Blazer, S.L. Health-Related Physical Fitness: Concepts and Activities for Elementary School Children. Edina, MN: Burgess International Group Inc.

CHAPTER 2

DEFINITION AND DESCRIPTION
OF SPORT AEROBICS

Aerobic exercise can be described as continuous rigorous activity lasting beyond two minutes and utilizing the large muscles of the body. It conditions the heart by temporarily increasing the body's use of oxygen for the production of energy. The heart eventually adjusts to this demand and so is able to transport oxygen more efficiently to the muscles, thereby increasing their capacity to do work. There are three basic principles which must be adhered to in an aerobic workout. These are: intensity, duration and frequency.

Intensity refers to the stressfulness of the activity. It is generally expressed as a percentage of maximum heart rate (the number of times the heart can beat in one minute). Research has indicated that heart rate should be maintained at 60-85 percent of maximum heart rate throughout the exercise period in order for cardiorespiratory improvements to occur. A simple formula for determining an individual's desired exercise heart rate range is shown in Figure 2.1.

```
[(220-age) - RHR] x .60 + RHR = lower end of range
[(220-age) - RHR] x .85 + RHR = upper end of range
              (RHR = Resting Heart Rate)
```

FIGURE 2.1: Formula for desired exercise heart rate.

To measure heart rate, the pulse may be taken by palpating either the radial artery at the base of the thumb at the temporal artery in front of the ear. A convenient method for taking the pulse is to use a ten second count and then multiply by six. The total is the number of heartbeats per minute.

Duration is the amount of time spent per exercise session. Five to 30 minutes is generally sufficient, depending upon the intensity of the activity and individual levels of fitness.

The third principle is frequency, or the number of exercise sessions per week. Participation in an aerobic program at least three days per week is necessary for cardiorespiratory fitness to improve. Six days a week is maximum. It is important to give the body at least one day a week for rest and recovery.

MEANING OF SPORT SPECIFIC

As a fitness activity, sport aerobics combines physical exercise with sport specific skills. The routines are designed to increase the heart's ability to pump blood more efficiently throughout the body, while at the same time improving one's level of skill-related fitness. The general components of skill-related fitness are: agility, balance, coordination, power, reaction time and speed.

The term sport specific refers to those movements which are geared toward a particular skill activity. Training for a particular sport in no way guarantees that the level of fitness, or degree of skill achieved will be adequate for other sports. This is because exercise produces both muscular and neuromuscular adaptations in relation to the movement pattern being performed. The nerve pathways become more efficient with continued repetition, but only with respect to the specific skill activity. Practice must therefore be related to the dominant features of the skill itself. In order words, specificity means relating the unique physical requirements of a sport to a practice patterns that will elicit the exact biological responses that produce the skill.

Rhythm and Sport Skills

The human body is inherently rhythmic. Many physiological functions such as breathing and the beating of the heart occur in regular, recurring patterns requiring no conscious effort or control. Similarly, any bodily movement will produce a distinct rhythmic pattern in the ebb and flow of muscular energy. The relative duration of individual muscular actions, as well as when they begin and end with respect to one another, is often sensed rather than measured or counted in any way. However, sport skill development is dependent upon the ability to give conscious rhythmic form and structure to a complex movement sequence. Musical accompaniment for sport routines enhances sensory awareness of physical rhythms by allowing movement to occur in direct response to a steady recurrent beat.

Endurance and Sport Skills

All sports call for endurance. Even those sports which are primarily anaerobic in nature require a certain level of cardio-respiratory fitness before they can be mastered. The term anaerobic refers to any vigorous activity lasting less than two to three minutes. Anaerobic activities involves an all-out burst of muscle effort and relies on chemical reactions inside the body (rather than oxygen) for the production of energy. Many popular sports such as basketball, football and tennis are considered anaerobic because they involve frequent stopping and starting. Due to the tremendous physical demands anaerobic exercise makes on the body, individuals should be careful not to engage in this type of activity until they are aerobically fit. The development of cardiorespiratory endurance is paramount to the ability to perform strenuous exercise without excessive fatigue.

10

BENEFITS OF SPORT AEROBICS

Cardiorespiratory endurance is the fitness of the heart, lungs and blood vessels, which together comprise the body's oxygen transport system. The efficient utilization of oxygen for energy is dependent upon three factors. These are: the ability to rapidly breathe large amounts of air, the ability to forcefully deliver large volumes of blood, and the ability to effectively deliver oxygen to all parts of the body.

Improving Endurance

Cardiorespiratory endurance may be improved through a program of regular aerobic exercise. The heart responds to this type of exercise by developing a greater capacity to pump more oxygenated blood throughout the body with fewer contractions and less effort. This enables the body to more efficiently supply the working muscle with energy, and to increase the elimination of metabolic waste products, thus delaying the onset of fatigue. Optimal cardiorespiratory endurance is also associated with a decreased risk of coronary heart disease. This disease affects the arteries that supply blood to the heart muscle itself. It is responsible for over one half of all American deaths each year.

Other Physiological Changes

In addition to improving cardiorespiratory endurance, participation in a sport aerobics program may produce a number of other physiological changes relating to total body fitness. These include the following:

1. Less chance of developing high blood pressure through improved circulation.
2. Maintenance of proper body weight due to improved fat metabolism and increased caloric expenditure.
3. Increase of muscle strength and endurance.
4. Increased flexibility.
5. Regulation of adrenal secretions resulting in a greater resistance to emotional stress.
6. A more regular elimination of solid wastes.
7. Possible delay in the aging process.

Secondary Benefits

Possible secondary benefits include improved physical appearance and self-esteem. Although hard to quantify, these factors may contribute to enhanced psychological functioning.

A final benefit of sport aerobics is that sport skill development may progress at a faster rate. As mentioned previously, neuromuscular control becomes more efficient with continued repetition of a specific sport skill activity. In addition, an increased level of fitness with regard to endurance, body weight, muscle strength and flexibility lessens the possibility that inefficient movement habits will be established due to fatigue. Because many injuries are the result of fatigue, the chance of injury is therefore reduced.

SUMMARY

Sport aerobics is a fitness activity which combines aerobic exercise with the development of sport skills. Aerobic exercise conditions the cardiorespiratory system by requiring oxygen for the production of energy. Sport skill development is dependent upon repeated practice of the unique physical requirements needed for a particular sport activity. There are several criteria which must be present in a sport aerobics program. These are:

1. Heart rate should be maintained at 60-85 percent of maximum heart rate throughout the exercise period.
2. The movement must be continuous for a duration of 5-30 minutes.
3. Participation must occur at least three days per week.
4. Practice must be related to the dominant features of the particular skill activity.
5. The movements must be given a conscious rhythmic form and structure.
6. A minimum level of fitness is required prior to participation.

The primary benefit of participation in a sport aerobics program is improved cardiorespiratory endurance. This means that the body is able to more efficiently supply the working muscles with energy. It is also associated with a decreased risk of coronary heart disease. Many of the physiological changes that occur with sport aerobics contribute to improvements in total body fitness and also allow sport skill development to progress at a faster rate.

SELECTED BIBLIOGRAPHY

Kisselle, J., and Mazzeo, K. Aerobic Dance: A Way to Fitness. Englewood, CO: Morton Publishing Co., 1983.

McGlynn, G. Dynamics of Fitness: A Practical Approach. Dubuque, IA: Wm. C. Brown Publishers, 1982.

Petray, C.K., and Blazer, S.L. Health-Related Physical Fitness: Concepts and Activity for Elementary School Children. Edina, N.Y.: Bellwether Press, 1986.

Shell, C.G., ed. The Dancer As Athlete. Champaign, ILL: Human Kinetics Publishers, Inc., 1986.

CHAPTER 3

SELECTED SKILLS FOR THE ROUTINES

There are basic skills unique to each sport activity. There are also many skills that carry over from one sport to another. Skills related to sports are either sport specific or basic in nature. In the development and use of sport specific aerobic routines, it is important to have the appropriate skills choreographed to good music. Often the decision on which skills to use is not an easy one to make. It is important to remember that basic motor skills (walking, running, jumping, throwing, etc.) are used in practically all sports and not unique to any particular one. On the other hand, each sport has skills unique to it.

The material in this chapter deals with the selection of sport related skills that can be used in aerobic routines. The emphasis will be upon analyzing the sport, selecting appropriate skills, and sequencing the skills. This material is presented to help the reader either develop sport specific aerobic routines or modify and change the ones listed in this text. Modification or change is often needed to meet specific needs.

ANALYZING THE SPORT

To develop good sport aerobic routines, it is necessary to analyze the sport for which the routines are to be developed. At this stage it is not an analysis of a single sport skill, but rather an analysis of the sport as to what skills are required for participation. Every sport requires an individual to have certain skills for successful participation. These skills are classified into one of two categories which are basic motor skills and sport specific skills. Both categories must be considered and examined closely as routines are developed.

Basic Motor Skills

Basic motor skills have a certain amount of carry over from one sport to another. Nonetheless, these skills are necessary, if there is to be good execution of the sport specific skills. Many times individuals put sport specific skills before the development of basic motor skills. Developing the ability to consistently and effectively execute selected sport skills does not happen in this manner.

Basic motor skills must be identified and listed as related to a specific sport. One way to do this is by using the chart shown in Figure 3.1.

Sport _____			
*Put a (x) in the appropriate column.			
Basic Motor Skills	**Important**	**Very Important**	**Critical**
Balancing			
Running			
Walking			
Jumping			
Hopping			
Throwing			
Catching			
Kicking			
Others:			
1.			
2.			
3.			

FIGURE 3.1   Chart for analyzing basic motor skills.

Sport specific routines are developed to make use of basic motor skills as related to the selected sport. Therefore, it is important to identify which skills are most often used when participating in the sport itself. For example, running would be "critical" for soccer routines. "Balancing" is critical to all sports. "Jumping" is more "critical" to basketball and volleyball than for soccer. The analysis of a sport to identify basic motor skills used in the activity is not a difficult task but a critical one. When all parts of a sport specific routine start to take shape, it will be obvious that basic motor skills are used as much or more than the sport specific skills. It is the basic motor skills that make for an easy transition from one sport specific skill to another.

Sport Specific Skills

Sport specific skills are somewhat different from basic motor skills. These skills are the specific movements needed to participate in a given sport. The rules of a sport may dictate, to some extent, what these movements are to be. These skills may also be nothing more than an extension of a basic motor skill with more complex movement. For example, kicking is a basic motor skill in soccer and a sport specific skill as well. The execution of each is different. The analysis of a sport to determine the specific skills may be done by using the process described in Figure 3.2

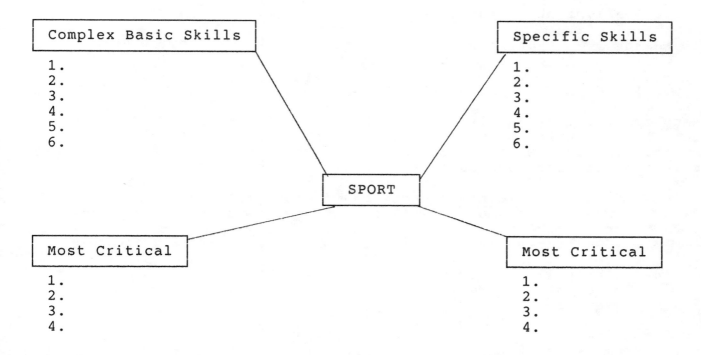

FIGURE 3.2 Process for identifying skills specific to a sport.

There may be more than six skills for each category or more than four that are critical. Identifying the skills that are "critical" is just a means of making sure important skills are not left out. With any sport, it is necessary to ask the following question: What are the most critical skills that an individual needs to know for active participation in a given sport? These are the skills that become the main focus of a routine. It is entirely possible to develop a single routine around one or two specific skills. The most effective routines are those that have a good mix of basic motor skills with sport specific skills.

SELECTING AND SEQUENCING THE APPROPRIATE SKILLS

Once all of the skills related to sport have been identified, the next step is to select and sequence the movements into a routine format. Some sport related skills do not work well in the routines because the movements required are less than aerobic in nature. The skills that do not require movement which is aerobic can be used in the routines but would affect the desired outcome. The selection and sequencing phase is the part of the process where the movements required for various skills are combined as an aerobic exercise.

Selecting the Skills

It is best to select those skills that require movements to be completed in an even four count sequence. For example, kicking a soccer ball might follow this pattern:

Ready   Bring Foot   Forward Kick   Follow Through
               and Leg Back

1   2   3   4

Many sport related skills follow this type of pattern. Skills that do
not follow this pattern will be more difficult to choreograph to
music. The following guidelines can be used to select the most appropriate skills for developing an aerobic routine.

1. Count the <u>movement sequence</u> of each skill.
2. Use basic motor skills that have a good <u>flow</u> with the
    specific skills.
3. Use those skills that are most often used in <u>game like</u>
    conditions.
4. The skill should have <u>aerobic</u> type movements.
5. The skill should be <u>easy</u> to perform with or without
    equipment.

The consideration given to each of the preceding guidelines should
vary from sport to sport. It is necessary to keep the nature of the
sport in mind during this process. Basketball is more aerobic in
nature than football, therefore it is likely that basketball skills
will be easier to select for aerobic routines than will football
skills.

Sequencing the Skills

    The movements in a routine should be sequenced in such a way that
the effort required to execute them is aerobic. An example of this
is: running in place for 16 beats, then run in place dribbling a
basketball for 16 beats, and then run in place dribbling a basketball
for seven beats, passing on the 8th beat. It is not a good idea to
format a routine so that dribbling and running comes before the
running phase. The sequence of this movement example is starting with
a basic motor skill (running) and progresses to the sport specific
skills of dribbling and passing.
    After deciding which skills to use in a routine, it is important
to follow these guidelines for getting the movements in proper
sequence.

1. The <u>transition</u> from one skill to another should be
    smooth and easy for the participant.
2. The movements of each skill must be in a <u>direct sequence</u>
    to the music selected.
3. Use the basic motor skill as a <u>lead-up</u> to the sport
    specific skill.
4. The sequence of all movements should be as near <u>game-
    like</u> as possible.
5. The skills should be in an order that allows for maximum
    <u>aerobic</u> movement.

Sequencing skills for an aerobic routine is much like telling a story. There is a beginning, a middle and an end. For the story to read well, there must be good flow. The same is true with routines. The movement flow must be good in order to obtain the maximum potential for an aerobic workout.

The sequencing of skills is a fun experience. At this point one gets to test creative skills and talents for matching selected movements to music. Much of this process is trial and error. It is possible to select certain skills for a routine and it will not work. For whatever reasons, the movements of the skills cannot be matched with music. When this happens, drop the skills and the music and start over. Select new skills and new music, if needed. Generally, a new routine can be developed at this point.

Another problem, usually minor in nature, associated with sequencing skills is that the finished product will be too easy or too difficult. It is entirely possible to make a routine too complex or simple for the participants. When this happens a simple change or modification will solve the problem. The following trouble spots should be checked for a possible change or modification.

1. Order of skills in relation to game-like situations.
2. Movements too fast or slow for the music.
3. Too much stopping of movement.
4. Movements are in a simple to complex order.
5. Elements of excitement and fun present.

Sequencing should be viewed as a challenge to put movements in such an order that participants get aerobic exercise and practice sports skills in one experience.

SUMMARY

Selecting basic motor skills and sport specific skills is an important part of the total process for developing sport aerobic routines. There are countless ways in which these skills could be used to develop good routines. This makes for good variety in aerobic routines of this nature.

The selection of skills for aerobic routines involves analyzing the sport. It is important to know and identify all skills that are required to participate in a given sport activity. The analysis must identify both basic motor skills and sport specific skills. There are guidelines that can be followed to make this part of the process relatively easy.

The sequencing of the movements for the different skills is one of the more challenging parts of the total process. It is during this stage that skills selected must be considered for a particular piece of music. The creative thought process can certainly be used in the sequencing phase.

Selecting and sequencing skills is vital to the development of sport specific aerobic routines. Going through this process properly can insure the development of routines that have good flow and smooth transitions from beginning to end.

17

SUGGESTED ACTIVITIES

1. Select your favorite sport. Using the charts in Figures 3.1 and 3.2, identify and classify the skills used in this sport. Do the same with your least favorite sport.

2. Using the skills identified in first exercise, select a few of the skills from each category. Now determine whether or not the movements in these skills can be executed to an even four count beat. If not, what could be done to make the movements appropriate for a four count sequence.

3. Take two to four skills and sequence them to a rhythmical pattern. Is the flow of the movements good? If not, try to determine why and make changes accordingly.

SELECTED BIBLIOGRAPHY

Harris, J.A., Pittman, A.M. and Waller, M.S. Dance a While. (6th ed). New York, NY: MacMillan Publishing Company, 1988.

Thomas, J.R. and Nelson, J.K. Introductions to Research in Health, Physical Education, Recreation, and Dance. Champaign, ILL: Human Kinetics Publishers, Inc., 1985.

Sage, G.H. Introduction to Motor Behavior: A Neuropsychological Approach (2nd). Reading, MASS: Addison-Wesley Publishing Company, 1977.

Seefeldt, V. (Ed). Handbook for Youth Sports Coaches. Reston, VA: AAHPERD, 1987.

CHAPTER 4

DEVELOPMENT OF ROUTINES

The primary purpose of any sport specific aerobic routine is to integrate the basic principles of cardiorespiratory fitness with the development of sport specific skills. For a routine to be considered aerobic, the heart rate must be maintained at a targeted level of intensity for an extended period of time. This type of workout requires continuous movement, utilizing all of the major muscle groups. With regard to the development of sport skill, each routine should provide participants with the necessary opportunity to learn movement techniques which can be applied to a future sport situation.

DEVELOPING A FORMAT

There are three points to consider when developing the format of each routine. These are: movement content, progression, and pacing. In terms of movement content, it is advisable to target one particular type of skill upon which to build each routine. A routine which probes different aspects of a single skill is better than one that tries to cover a lot of material superficially. Participants will not become bored so long as they are challenged by new considerations. A routine which is centered around a single skill will not necessarily lack variety of movement. You can exhaust the possibility of the material by breaking each skill down into its most fundamental locomotor steps, floor patterns and body movements. Analyze each activity accurately and decide what particular technical controls can be stressed in order to prevent the establishment of careless movement habits. Try to anticipate possible errors in execution and ways to avoid or correct them. Formulate a clear idea of exactly what the level of skill performance should be as a result of the routine.

Content and Progression

The exact selection of movement experiences for a routine should allow for progression towards a minimum standard of accomplishment. Begin each routine with simple, familiar movements that can be performed with assurance. Teaching a complex movement series all at once can slow down the pace of the class due to the extra time required for explanations. It can be especially frustrating, if one is unfamiliar with the skill activity or does not learn it quickly. A satisfying progression is one which builds to a climax by advancing from the simple to the complex. Keep in mind first establishing a specific locomotor step before adding the floor patterns or arm movement. In general, the order of progression should be determined by the relationship of the familiar movement used as a point of departure to the skill being developed. Build the movement material so that each new experience is logically related to the one preceding it.

Pacing

    A final point to consider when developing the format of your routine is pacing. As stated previously, <u>continuous movement</u> is necessary for keeping the routine aerobic in nature. However, any movement can become exhausting if repeated or maintained at the same intensity for too long. Energy expenditure must be organized to accommodate variety. Recognizing this need is essential for preventing over-fatigue and reducing the risk of injury.
    Pacing can be achieved by alternating high intensity, vigorous movement with one that is less strenuous or that works a different set of muscles. Combining activities such as running and jumping with one like walking allows for some slowing down without actually stopping. Similarly, the body can get needed muscle rest very quickly by changing from one part to another, as when working one side of the body and then the other.
    Dynamic contrasts can also be achieved by means of adjustments in the size of a movement and the number of muscle groups used. Large movements which cover much space tend to increase workout intensity, as does movement involving both the upper and lower body.

SELECTING THE MUSIC

    Selecting music which corresponds to your movement needs is requisite to good choreography. Different types of music elicit different senses of movement, not all of which are suitable for aerobic routines.
    All music has a particular rhythmical structure in relation to time and energy. In order to determine this pattern of organization, both time and energy must be measured. The basic unit that measures time is known as the beat. It is a steady, recurring pulse which can be heard or felt consistently throughout a piece of music.

Beat, Meter and Tempo

    Beats are grouped into measures by the regular occurrence of accented beats. The accented beat is stronger than the other beats in the measure due to the placement of additional force or emphasis. A measure may contain any number of beats, provided that the sense of grouping is not last.
    Meter refers to the organization of measures within a piece of music to form a certain underlying rhythm. Three common rhythms are listed. These are divided into measures, as indicated by the / mark. The heavy accent of each rhythm is indicated by the symbol "'". Each example consists of four measures (Figure 4.1).

```
EXAMPLE   2/4:  1' 2 / 1' 2 / 1' 2 / 1' 2
EXAMPLE   4/4:  1' 2 3 4 / 1' 2 3 4 / 1' 2 3 4 / 1' 2 3 4
EXAMPLE   3/4:  1' 2 3 / 1' 2 3 / 1' 2 3 / 1' 2 3
```

FIGURE 4.1:   Examples of three common rhythms
and how each is organized.

When listening or moving to music, there is a natural tendency to
follow the accented beats. For this reason, it is wise to avoid music
with complex rhythmical structures such as frequent changes in meter,
melodies which begin and end in the middle of a measure, or two
rhythms occurring simultaneously. Selecting music with a steady beat
that can be clearly heard or felt will avoid confusion for both you
and your participants.

Another aspect of rhythm to consider is the tempo, or speed. The
underlying beat can be fast, slow or of moderate tempo, each of which
influences the quality of the music. Slower tempos tend to evoke
feelings of relaxation, or even lethargy. Faster tempos tend to
create feelings of excitement and exhilaration, indicative of an
increased sense of vitality. A moderate tempo is one which falls
somewhere in between these two points.

Choreographing

When choreographing movement to music, it is necessary to determine when a slow tempo becomes moderate, and moderate becomes fast.
In other words, fast is faster than what? A good rule of thumb to
follow for estimating moderate tempo is to relate it to the rate of
normal walking. Since one aim of sport specific aerobics is to maintain an elevated heart rate, moderate to fast tempos are preferable.

With these elements of rhythm in mind, musical choices are clearer
but there is still a wide selection to consider. Many instructors
limit themselves to contemporary or popular music because it is easily
accessible, and familiar to almost everyone. Other types of music one
may wish to consider are: country, bluegrass, motown, sixties rock
and roll, and movie sound tracks. Many broadway show tunes, written
especially to be danced to, lend themselves particularly well to
aerobic routines. Here again, variety is important. The music that
you select can be your best motivator for maintaining interest and
participation. Even after a routine has been choreographed, it does
not always have to be performed to the same song. Periodically
changing the music for a particular routine can help to avoid
monotony. Finally, it is important to make musical choices that you
enjoy. You will be hearing them a lot, first as you choreograph, and
later when you are teaching.

DEVELOPING THE ROUTINE

Once you have selected the music you wish to use for a particular routine, listen to it several times. Be sure that you can follow not only the steady beat, but also the basic rhythm. This can be accomplished by clapping or even writing down each beat. Count the beats in sets of four or eight if possible. You will want to choreograph to these counted sets of beats rather than to the melody. The only time the melody becomes important to choreography is when it repeats itself and you wish to do the same movement sequence each time. For example, you can perform the same step pattern each time the chorus is repeated.

Preparation of Routine

In preparing each routine, the overall pattern of movement should be worked out in detail. Decide which aspects of the skill you wish to focus upon. Plan to include at least two, but no more than four different movement sequences. This will provide enough variety to keep the routine interesting, yet still easy to learn and remember. For example, if you are choreographing a basketball dribbling routine, you might choose to emphasize different locomotor steps. One movement sequence might incorporate running, another sliding, and a third pivoting. Remember to arrange the movement sequences in an order which allows the routine to build to a climax.

Establish step patterns first and coordinate those with the music, then coordinate the arms or other gestures (movement of any non-weight bearing body part) with the steps. Few movement rhythms are actually as simple and regular as the musical beat itself. Any number of different rhythms can be created by combining or dividing the beats into time intervals of various lengths. When the time intervals are all of the same length (all slow or all quick), the movement rhythm is even. Fundamental locomotor steps which fall into this category are: walking, running, leaping, jumping and hopping. Because these steps are familiar to almost everyone, their manner of performance is often taken for granted.

Developing Steps for the Music

There are several ways steps can be set to music. Some possible arrangements are (Figure 4.2):

4/4	step	step	step	step	walking or running
	R	L	R	L	step pattern
	___	___	___	___	rhythm pattern
					underlying beat
	1	2	3	4	counts

4/4	step		step		walking
	R		L		step pattern
	_____		_____		rhythm pattern
					underlying beat
	1	2	3	4	counts

4/4	step	step	step	step	step	step	step	step	running
	R	L	R	L	R	L	R	L	step pattern
	___	___	___	___	___	___	___	___	rhythm pattern
									underlying beat
	1	&	2	&	3	&	4	&	counts

FIGURE 4.2: Possible arrangements for movement to 4/4 music.

When the time intervals are not of all the same value, but are any combination of slow and quick, the movement rhythm is uneven. Some fundamental steps which form an uneven rhythm are skipping, sliding, galloping, and the twostep. These (Figure 4.3) must also be performed in relation to the beat of the music:

4/4	step	hop	step	hop	step	hop	step	hop	skipping
	R	R	L	L	R	R	L	L	step pattern
	___	__	___	__	___	__	___	__	rhythm pattern
									underlying beat
	1	&	ah	2	&	ah	3	&	ah	4	&	ah	counts

4/4	step	close	step		two-step
	R	L	R		step pattern
	___	___	_____		rhythm pattern
					underlying beat
	1	2	3	4	counts

FIGURE 4.3: Possible arrangements for movement when steps form an uneven ryhthm

In terms of dynamics, the effect of timing on movement must not be overlooked. Keep in mind that as the tempo of a movement sequence increases, you will need to take smaller steps and cover less space.

Attention must also be given to accents of execution. Energy is required for the performance of any movement, but the amount may vary according to the movement and the manner in which it is performed. An accent of execution is the result of a sudden increase in the use of energy. Many movement patterns contain innate accents of execution, usually performed unconsciously. For example, in sports involving the projection of an object, such as a ball, an accent of execution will naturally occur as force is imparted from the body to the ball.

Ease of movement is facilitated when accents of execution are timed to coincide with the beats of the music. To illustrate this point, jump up and down several times, making contact with the floor on each beat. Repeat the jumps, but change the timing so that you are in the air on the beat. If performed accurately, the first set of jumps will occur as a direct response to the beat, requiring less conscious effort.

Writing the Routine

Write down the routine as you work out each sequence. Decide how many times each step will be performed, and the number of beats required for this. Most of the routines in this book repeat a particular step pattern two, four, eight, or 16 times. You want just enough repetition to make the routine easy to remember without becoming boring. Difficult step patterns will generally require more repetition than simpler ones in order for participants to feel comfortable with the movement. Be sure to work both sides of the body equally. Muscular balance is important for reducing susceptibility to injury. If a movement sequence primarily uses muscles on one side of the body, it will need to be performed an equal number of times on the opposite side.

Each routine does not need to last as long as the song. The entire routine or any portion of it may be repeated until the music ends.

EVALUATING FOR CONTINUOUS MOVEMENT

For a sport routine to be considered aerobic, movement must begin with the onset of the music and continue non-stop until the song is over. The step patterns must be connected to the music and also to one another so as to be performed with any interruptions or breaks.

Practice Performing the Routine

The best way to evaluate a routine for continuous movement is to practice performing it to the music. Make certain that the choreography actually coincides with the tempo and the number of beats allotted for each step pattern. Be aware of any nuances in phrasing, such as musical retards. These can generally be compensated for by extending the size of the movement to cover more space. If the music should contain any odd sections, or extra beats, these will need to be filled in with additional movement.

Carefully examine how different steps have been combined. Pay particular attention to the techniques of "getting into" a step or "getting out" of it. Make sure that the transitions from one step pattern to another are logical. Awkward or difficult transitions can be confusing and disrupt the flow of movement. Whenever possible, choreograph your steps so that they may begin on either foot. In routines where a directional pattern does influence the foot relationship, establish a rule that each new pattern will begin on the right foot.

Alternate Movements

When teaching a routine, instruct participants to keep moving no matter what. Jumping or running in place can always be substituted for specific footwork, if one has trouble with a particular step pattern. Maintaining an elevated heart rate is ultimately more important than exacting technique. To determine if the routine is aerobically challenging, check your pulse after performing it and see if you have reached your targeted level of intensity.

KNOWING THE SKILLS FOR ROUTINE DEVELOPMENT

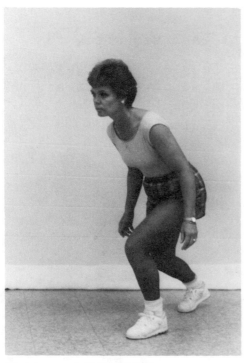

Stance and Eye Position

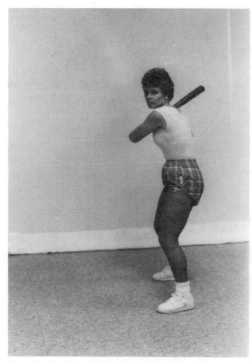

Good Body Alignment

SUMMARY

Improvement in cardiovascular endurance and technical skill through sport specific aerobics will be missed unless there is a constant challenge to work at full capacity. The choreographic process requires advanced preparation, with a complete understanding of how movement is consciously given form and rhythmic structure to achieve its goals. The following guidelines will help when choreographing sport aerobic routines:

1. Select one particular type of skill upon which to build each routine. Exhaust the possibility of your material by breaking each skill down into its most fundamental components.

2. Allow for progression towards a minimum standard of accomplishment. Build the routine to a climax by advancing from the simple to complex.

3. Do not overwork a strenuous activity. Pace the routine by alternating high intensity movement with one that is less demanding or uses a different set of muscles.

4. Choose music with a consistent beat and a moderate to fast tempo.

5. Include enough variety of movement in the routine to keep it interesting, yet easy to remember.

6. Establish step patterns first and coordinate those with the music before adding arms or other gestures.

7. Coordinate any accents of execution to coincide with the beats of the music.

8. Write down the routine as you work out each sequence.

9. Practice performing the routine to music. Make sure that the movement is continuous and also of sufficient intensity to be aerobically challenging.

SUGGESTED ACTIVITIES

1. Select a particular sport skill and develop four different move-
    ment sequences from it. Include both high and low intensity
    movement. Arrange the movement sequences in an order which allows
    for progression from the simple to the more complex.

2. Find three different pieces of music which might be considered
    appropriate for a sport aerobic routine. Identify the meter of
    each song, and practice clapping to the steady beat. Counting in
    sets of eight, practice walking or running in place to the beat of
    each song.

3. Select a simple step pattern and determine whether the movement
    rhythm is even or uneven. Coordinate the step pattern to music
    using counts. Time any accents of execution to coincide with the
    beats of the music.

SELECTED BIBLIOGRAPHY

Hayes, E. An Introduction to the Teaching of Dance. New York, N.Y.:
    Ronald Press Co., 1964.

Humphrey, D. The Art of Making Dances. New York, N.Y.: Rinehart and
    Co., Inc., 1959.

Kiselle, J., M.Ed. and Mazzeo, K.S., M.Ed. Aerobic Dance: A Way to
    Fitness. Englewood, CO: Morton Publishing, Co., 1983.

Wilmoth, S.K. Leading Aerobic Dance Exercise. Champaign, IL: Human
    Kinetics, 1986.

BASKETBALL

Basketball is an activity enjoyed by many people of different ages and various skill levels. It is such a universal game that some people play it for fun, while others play for the exercise, and yet, others may play for the challenge and love of the sport. Basketball seems to be such a popular activity, because it offers immediate reinforcement. One simply makes a basket and the reward is immediate. Some success is enjoyed very quickly, which motivates an individual to play or try it again. As a result, it becomes a form of exercise!

BASKETBALL AND FITNESS

In recent years, there seems to have been a steady increase of participants in basketball related activities. Some of this may be due to the increased emphasis upon cardiovascular fitness. Basketball is certainly a strenuous activity and does tax the cardiorespiratory system of the participants, if correctly played.

Basketball Skills

The skills required to adequately participate in a game of basketball (modified or official) are complex to say the least. Most all basketball related skills require an individual to execute a sequence of movements in a rhythmical manner. Many of the skills are an outgrowth of basic motor skills, therefore the refinement process of the skills should include use of the basic skills.

Strength and Endurance

Strength and endurance are very important qualities to have, if basic basketball skills are to be executed properly. The same may be said as these qualities relate to basic motor skill execution. As an individual develops or refines his/her basketball skills, the refinement of the basic motor skills also occurs. Aerobic routines designed around basketball skills will likely have more effect on endurance than on strength, but logically one quality tends to reinforce or compliment the other.

BASKETBALL ROUTINES

Fifteen sport aerobic routines for promoting aerobic fitness and developing or refining basketball skills have been developed. The routines were developed with emphasis on basic basketball skills as listed in Figure 5.1.

1.	Passing	6.	Shooting
2.	Pivoting	7.	Ball Handling
3.	Defensive Sliding	8.	Rebounding
4.	Running and Jogging	9.	Catching
5.	Jumping	10.	Balance and Body Control

FIGURE 5.1. Basic basketball skills for which
the routines are developed.

Each routine can easily be modified or changed to meet specific needs as dictated by the skill or age levels of the participants. Music other than that suggested may be used. A music change may require the movements be choreographed differently than that described. Changes in routines or music should not create problems as long as the flow of movement is good.

These routines can be used with all ages. Basketball skill levels and fitness levels would be better criteria for determining which to use with a particular age group. Continuous movement is a critical factor, if the participant is to receive cardiorespiratory benefits from the experience.

USE OF IMAGERY AND SKILL EXECUTION

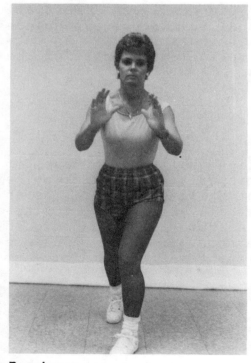

Passing

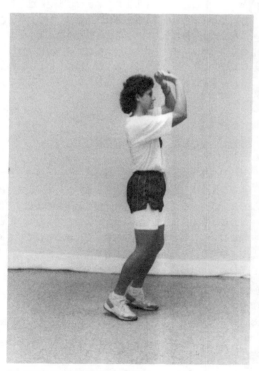

Shooting Without Ball

BASKETBALL

SKILLS: Defense (guarding), Bounce, Passing and Pivoting

SUGGESTED MUSIC: "Physical" (Olivia-Newton John)

EQUIPMENT: Basketballs or other balls that bounce. Should have enough for one-half of the group.

PARTS	BEATS	MOVEMENT	DESCRIPTION
1	8	Guard/slide step.	Go to left.
2	8	Guard/slide step.	Go to right.
3	8	Guard/forward.	Forward.
4	4	Pivot/bounce pass.	Pass on last beat.
5	4	Jog.	Jog in place.
6		Repeat all parts.	

Repeat the routine until end of music.

INSTRUCTIONS:

Balls are given to one-half of the group. Participants without a ball start the routine on defense guarding a partner using a sliding step. When the pivot is made and a bounce pass follows, partners change from offense to defense and vice versa. Emphasis should be upon passing the ball to an individual who is open. It is not necessary for one partner to pass to another. If an open participant cannot be found, then the individual should keep the ball and continue through next sequence of the routine. To get the desired time for exercise, the music may be repeated.

BASKETBALL

SKILLS: Lay-ups

SUGGESTED MUSIC: "Crush on You" (Jet)

EQUIPMENT: Basketballs or balls that bounce. Should have
enough for one-half of the group.

PARTS	BEATS	MOVEMENT	DESCRIPTION
1	72	Jog in place. (chorus)	Clap hands to beat of music.
2	8	Four step-hops forward.	Two count step hop – begin with right foot.
	4	Skip back.	One skip per beat – begin with right foot.
	4	Skip.	Circle to right.
		Repeat Part 2.	
3	16	Run right, run left. Step-hop 1/4 turn left and repeat step beginning with the left.	Four counts each direction. Forming complete square alternating right and left to begin step.
	16	Repeat the above.	Make 1/4 turns to the right.
		Repeat Part 3	
4	32	Jog in place. (Chorus)	Clap hands to beat of music.
	16	Jog.	Form circle with groups and clap hands to beat of music.
	64	Repeat Part 3. (Verse) Omit the 1/4 turns.	Entire circle moves counter-clockwise.
5	32	Jog in place. (Chorus)	All face center of circle.
	48	Slide moving counter-clockwise in circle.	Clap hands to beat of music.

PARTS   BEATS   MOVEMENT   DESCRIPTION

          32   Jog in place.   All face center of circle.
                  (Chorus)

INSTRUCTIONS:

For remainder of the music run to pick up a basketball and begin
working with a partner taking turns dribbling and performing a layup
shot (as a pass) releasing the ball at the height of the step hop to
your partner moving in any direction. Be sure to work both left and
right sides. Simulate the proper lay-up techniques throughout the
routine extending the arm on the same side as knee joint is up on all
step-hops in the routine.

SKILLS FOR THE BASKETBALL ROUTINES

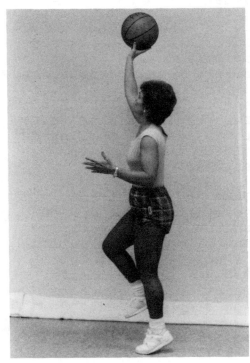

Lay-Up

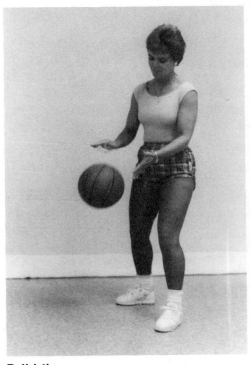

Dribbling

BASKETBALL

SKILLS: Passing, Dribbling, and Defensive Shuffling

SUGGESTED MUSIC: "Can You Feel It?" (Michael Jackson)

EQUIPMENT: Basketballs or balls that bounce. Should have enough for one half of the group.

PARTS	BEATS	MOVEMENT	DESCRIPTION
1	16	Move to right. Both ones and twos.	Ones take the balls and dribble moving right in a circle keeping the basketballs on the outside of the circle in right hands. Twos begin sliding to their right on the inside circle in a defensive shuffle position.
2	16	Jogging and passing.	Quick turn to face new partner and continue jogging but passing ball back and forth.
3	16	Move to left. Both ones and twos.	Ones take the balls and dribble moving left in a circle keeping the basketballs on the outside of the circle in left hands. Twos begin sliding to their left on the inside circle in defensive shuffle position.
4	8	Jogging steps to change position.	Ones and twos trade positions. Ones now on inside of circle facing out with twos on outside of circle facing in. Begin "jog and pass" maintaining constant non-stop movement.
5		Repeat the routine until end of music.	

INSTRUCTIONS:

Use a double circle formation with partners facing. Designate those on the outside of the circle (facing in) as ones (1s) and those on the inside circle (facing out) as twos (2s). Ones start the routine with a ball.

BASKETBALL

SKILLS: Dribbling and Ball Handling

SUGGESTED MUSIC: "Addicted to Love" (Robert Palmer)

EQUIPMENT: One basketball per participant.

PARTS	BEATS	MOVEMENT	DESCRIPTION
1	34	Stretching.	Leader directed. Holding ball.
2	32	Jog.	Raise ball low, middle, high, back to middle.
	16	Dribble - right hand.	Knees flexed, switch ball to left hand on 16th beat.
	16	Dribble - left hand.	Knees flexed, switch ball to right hand on 16th beat.
3	32	Jog.	Raise ball same as in Part 2.
	32	Body circles.	Circle body, ball at waist.
	16	Left leg circle.	Circle left leg, switch to right on 16th beat.
4	16	Right leg circle.	Circle right leg, switch on 16th beat.

Repeat the routine until end of music.

BASKETBALL

SKILLS: Passing

SUGGESTED MUSIC: "The Heat Is On" (Glenn Frey)

EQUIPMENT: None

PARTS	BEATS	MOVEMENT	DESCRIPTION
1	16	Jog.	In place.
2	8	Pass	Motion overhead pass while leaning forward. Make use of imagery.
3	16	Side slide 8 right, 8 left.	Side slide, clap to the right side slide, clap to the left for 16 beats.
4	8	Hop Kick.	Do four hop kicks alternating feet.

Repeat the routine until end of music.

INSTRUCTIONS:

It is advisable to double tape the music for more time to receive full benefits of the workout. Imagery is recommended for this routine.

BASKETBALL

SKILLS: Bounce Passing

SUGGESTED MUSIC: "Conga" (Miami Sound Machine)

EQUIPMENT: One basketball per circle (size of circle may vary).

PARTS	BEATS	MOVEMENT	DESCRIPTION
1	48	Slide step, bounce pass and catch.	Students slide clockwise in circle formation. Student with ball makes a bounce pass across the circle to somebody who catches the ball and does likewise.
2	48	Slide step, bounce pass and catch.	Circle changes to counterclockwise direction while still passing.
3	24	Slide step, bounce pass and catch.	Circle changes to clockwise. Leader adds another ball to each group.
	24	Slide step, bounce pass and catch.	Circle changes to counterclockwise movement.
4	32	Slide step, bounce pass and catch.	Circle changes to clockwise. Leader adds another ball to each group. Total of three balls per group. Circle changes to counterclockwise movement.

Repeat the routine until end of music.

BASKETBALL

SKILLS: Blocking and Pivoting

SUGGESTED MUSIC: "Rockin' at Midnight" (The Honeydrippers)

EQUIPMENT: None

PARTS	BEATS	MOVEMENT	DESCRIPTION
1	16	Run in place.	Sixteen running steps.
2	16	Block.	Jump with hands straight above head. Two beats per jump. Make eight blocks.
3	16	Run in place.	Sixteen running steps.
4	16	Pivot.	Two beats per pivot. Make eight pivots.

Repeat the routine until end of music.

INSTRUCTIONS:

Use imagery with the blocks. Participant pretending that he/she is blocking out offensive player after a shot.

BASKETBALL

SKILLS: Pivoting and Defense

SUGGESTED MUSIC: "Dancing in the Street" (Martha Reeves)

EQUIPMENT: None

PARTS	BEATS	MOVEMENT	DESCRIPTION
1	8	Pivots.	Class in scattered formation, planting one foot and turning with a step of the other foot.
2	16	Jogging.	Sixteen running steps.
3	4	Defensive position.	Keep body position low. Slide forward four counts, four counts back.
	4	Defensive position.	Slide forward four counts and backwards four counts.
		(Repeat Part 3, three times)	
4	16	Jog in place.	Sixteen running steps in place.
		Repeat the routine until end of music.	

INSTRUCTIONS:

It is advised to double tape the music or repeat the music in order to receive full benefits of the workout.

BASKETBALL

SKILLS: Jumping and Shuffling

SUGGESTED MUSIC: "Harden My Heart" (Quarter Flash)

EQUIPMENT: None

PARTS	BEATS	MOVEMENT	DESCRIPTION
1	16	Run.	In place, knees high, arms straight forward. Sixteen steps.
2	16	Shuffle.	Four counts forward, four backward, then side to side, right foot forward first time, left foot forward second time, then repeat.
3	4	Run.	In place, knees high, arms straight forward. Sixteen steps.
4	16	Jumps.	Two counts, jumping off your toes. Knees flexed, arms above your head.

Repeat the routine until end of music.

INSTRUCTIONS:

It is advised to double tape or repeat the music in order to receive full benefits of the workout.

BASKETBALL

SKILLS: Ball Handling and Dribbling

SUGGESTED MUSIC: "Would I Lie to You" (Eurythmics)

EQUIPMENT: Basketballs or a similar type of balls that will bounce. One ball per participant.

PARTS	BEATS	MOVEMENT	DESCRIPTION
1	16	Jump.	Alternate legs, holding the ball shoulder height or above.
	4	Pivot rest.	Two pivots on a two count. Make two pivots using two counts per pivot.
2	16	Ball handling.	Circle each leg twice, two counts per circle.
	4	Pivot rest.	Switch pivot foot, make two pivots two counts per pivot.
3	16	Dribbling.	Front and back, side to side, four dribbles per four counts. Hold the opposite hand up to protect the basketball from the defender.
	4	Pivot rest.	Switch pivot foot, make two, two counts per pivot.
4	16	Ball handling.	Figure eight twice using eight counts per time.
	4	Pivot rest.	Switch pivot foot, make two pivots, two counts per pivot.

Repeat the routine until end of music.

BASKETBALL

SKILLS: Dribbling, Passing, Catching, and Pivoting

SUGGESTED MUSIC: "Rockin the U.S.A." (John Cougar Mellencamp)

EQUIPMENT: Basketballs or similar type of balls that will bounce.
One ball per participants.

PARTS	BEATS	MOVEMENT	DESCRIPTION
1	16	Dribble.	Follow a line close to wall of gym, about six feet away. Take 16 dribbles, one per count.
2	16	Pass and catch.	Using a chest pass, pass the ball against the wall and catch it on the rebound. Do this four times, one pass and catch per two counts.
3	8	Pivots.	Two pivots, one per two counts.

Repeat the routine until end of music.

INSTRUCTIONS:

Instructor or leader may want to increase length of the music or use routine as a warm-up to other exercise.

BASKETBALL

SKILLS: Pivoting

SUGGESTED MUSIC: "Darlington County" (Bruce Springstein)

EQUIPMENT: None

PARTS	BEATS	MOVEMENT	DESCRIPTION
1	4	Jog forward.	Using four jogging steps.
	4	Pivot.	Make a circle using four steps off of a pivot.
	4	Jog backwards.	Use four jogging steps.
	4	Pivot.	Make a circle using four steps off of a pivot.
	16	Jumping jacks.	Four beats per completed movement. Do four one-half jumping jacks.

(Repeat Part 1, one time)

PARTS	BEATS	MOVEMENT	DESCRIPTION
2	16	Chest passes.	Two beats per pass and change directions. Use imagery, no equipment is needed.
	16	Jumping jacks.	Four beats per completed movement. Do four one-half jumping jacks.
	4	Pivot.	Make a circle using four steps off of a pivot. Clap hands to the feet.
	12	Jumping jacks.	Four beats per completed movement. Do three one half jumping jacks.

Repeat the routine until end of music.

INSTRUCTIONS:

For some of the movement, imagery is recommended.

BASKETBALL

<u>SKILLS</u>: Sliding and Pivoting

<u>SUGGESTED MUSIC</u>: "Thriller" (Michael Jackson)

<u>EQUIPMENT</u>: None

PARTS	BEATS	MOVEMENT	DESCRIPTION
1	8	Jog.	Taking jogging steps in different directions.
2	8	Pivot.	Make one complete circle, using two beats per pivot.
3	8	Jog.	
4	8	Slide step.	Two beats per sliding step. May move in any direction.

Repeat the routine until end of music.

<u>INSTRUCTIONS</u>:

Leader may want to use this routine as a warm-up to other exercises. Emphasis should be on correct pivots and sliding steps.

BASKETBALL

SKILLS: Ball Handling, Dribbling and Shooting

SUGGESTED MUSIC: "Boogie, Oogie Oogie"

EQUIPMENT: Basketballs or similar type of balls that will bounce.
One per participant.

PARTS	BEATS	MOVEMENT	DESCRIPTION
1	32	Shifting the ball.	Toss ball alternately from left to right hand.
2	8	Circle left leg.	Stride with left leg forward. Circle left leg four times and reverse direction four times.
	16	Figure eight both legs.	Weave ball through legs in figure eight fashion. Do eight times and reverse figure eight direction.
		(Repeat Part 1)	
3	8	Dribble.	With left hand.
	8	Dribble.	With right hand.
	16	Dribble.	Alternating left and right hands.
	8	Circle left leg.	Stride with left leg forward. Circle leg four times and reverse direction four times.
	8	Circle right leg.	Stride with right leg forward. Circle leg four times and reverse direction four times.
4	8	Dribble right moving at an angle – jump shot.	Don't release ball but pretend or imagine that shot was made.
	8	Dribble.	Backwards and shoot.

PARTS	BEATS	MOVEMENT	DESCRIPTION
	8	Dribble.	Forwards and shoot.
	8	Dribble.	Moving to the left at an angle and shoot.
	8	Dribble.	Moving to the right and shoot. Don't release the ball.
	8	Repeat dribble.	To the left.
	16	Repeat dribble.	To the right and to the left.

Repeat the routine until end of music.

INSTRUCTIONS:

Since this is a rather long routine, another option would be to do only Parts 1-2 and/or Parts 3-4 for duration of the music. This is advised, if participants are having difficulty learning all of the movements.

BASKETBALL

SKILLS: Slides and Pivots

SUGGESTED MUSIC: "Wanna Be Startin Somethin" (Michael Jackson)

EQUIPMENT: None

PARTS	BEATS	MOVEMENT	DESCRIPTION
1	32	Defensive slides.	Eight counts to each side from left to right with hands to the side in a defensive position. After each eight count, pivot on the left foot to face the opposite direction.
2	16	Eight pivots.	Pivot to the right and on the eighth count, step together.
3	16	Eight pivots.	Pivot to the left and on the eighth count, step together.
4	16	Four overhead passes and four chest passes.	Alternating overhead pass and chest pass, start with overhead pass and include jogging in place.

Repeat the routine until end of music.

INSTRUCTIONS:

In Part 1 it may be easier to do defensive slides for 16 beats going in one direction and then doing defensive slides for 16 beats in another direction.

SELECTED BIBLIOGRAPHY

Garrison, L. and Read, A. Fitness for Everybody. Palo Alto, CA: Mayfield Publishing Company, 1980.

Mazzeo, K. and Kisselle, J. Aerobic Dance. Englewood, CO: Morton Publishing Company, 1984.

Fox, R. Basketball. Englewood Cliffs, NJ: Prentice Hall, 1988.

Wilkes, G. Fundamentals of Coaching Basketball. Dubuque, IA: Wm. C. Brown Company Publishers, 1982.

SKILLS USED IN SOCCER ROUTINES

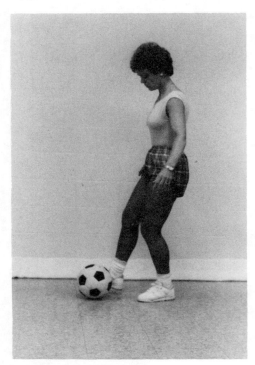

Instep Kick With Ball

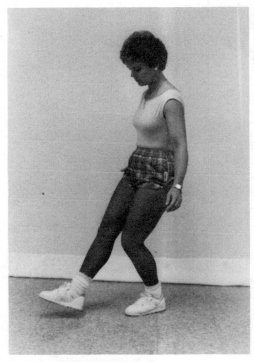

Instep Kick Without Ball

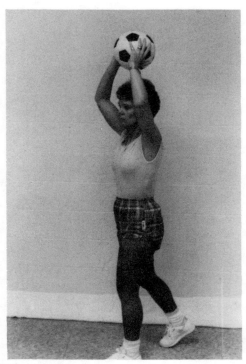

Throw In

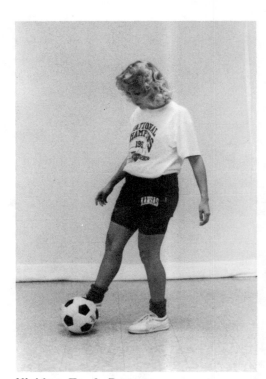

Kicking To A Partner

CHAPTER 6

SOCCER

Soccer is a game that obviously requires much use of the feet. Being able to maneuver the ball with the feet is necessary for the development of many soccer related skills (kicking, dribbling, shooting, etc.). For an individual to develop good soccer skills, the legs must receive some attention in the area of physical fitness. Since many aerobic exercises involve running, jogging, walking and other related movements, a healthy relationship seems to exist between soccer and physical fitness.

SOCCER AND FITNESS

In recent years, soccer has increasingly become one of the more popular sports among the younger segment of the population. The popularity of this sport maybe due to the fact that many can participate at one time and skill levels can vary without adverse effects. Another factor to consider as more people continue to participate in this sport is that it requires one to be active. Young people seem to be actively seeking sport games that provide a good aerobic type of workout. Soccer not only provides this type of experience, but also requires an individual to be physically fit in order to participate. The more physically fit he/she may be, the greater the chance of experiencing success in the execution of the skills.

Strength and Endurance

The game of soccer requires a lot of movement. The range of movement may vary from a jump and stretch to 30 yard sprint. When a sport requires this much movement, muscular strength and cardiovascular endurance are important factors when playing the game.

Lower body strength is critical because soccer requires much leg use from the participant. Such basic movement skills as running and jumping are often used to execute many soccer related skills. Upper body strength is also important. Soccer players often have to stretch, bend, and twist in order to execute other soccer skills. Soccer requires a good level of total body strength, if the participant is to experience success in playing the game. Both strength and endurance can be developed and maintained through proper exercise. Since soccer is like most any other sport, a specific type of fitness is required for proper skill execution.

SOCCER ROUTINES

Seventeen sport aerobic routines for soccer have been developed. These routines are designed to promote aerobic fitness and develop or refine an individual's soccer skills. The routines were designed around the basic skills listed in Figure 6.1

1. Dribbling	5. Heading
2. Throw-Ins	6. Basic Foot Movement
3. Kicking	7. Running
4. Trapping	8. Balancing

FIGURE 6.1 Basic soccer skills for which
the routines were developed.

Modification or changes in the movement can easily be changed on any of the routines. Skill and age levels of the participants should be considered a change or modification should be made. Music, other than that recommended, may also be used. A music change may require the movements to be choreographed differently than that described. When movement or music changes are made, it is important to keep a good movement flow.

These routines can be used with all ages. In selecting routines to be used the following should be considered: age, skill level, and fitness level. Once the movement in these routines starts, it is necessary for it to be continuous. Continuous movement is required in order for the participant to receive cardiorespiratory benefits from the experience.

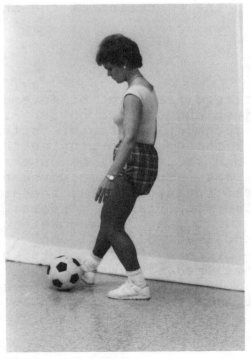

Moving With The Ball

SOCCER

SKILLS: Footwork and Dribbling

MUSIC: "Chase" (Soundtrack from Midnight Express)

EQUIPMENT: Soccer balls for one-half of the group.

PARTS	BEATS	MOVEMENT	DESCRIPTION
1	16	Hold.	Place ball on ground between partners. Get in ready position, holding hands.
2	8	Jumping to the right.	Jump per beat, moving around the ball holding hands with partner.
	8	Jumping to the left.	Jump per beat, moving around the ball holding hands with partner.
3	8	Jog backward four, jog forward four.	Moving away from the ball and then back to ball clapping on beats four and eight.
4	8	Cross step right (grapevine step). Cross step left.	Moving away from ball and back to ball clapping on beats four and eight. Four steps right and four steps left.
5	16	Partner one dribbles (instep) any direction then passes to partner two (two jogs along).	Dribble per beat keeping close control – pass on last four counts.
	16	Partner two dribbles (instep) any direction then gets ball in ready position (one jog along).	Dribble per beat keeping close control – get ball in ready position last four counts between partners.
6	16	Toe touches on ball with partner.	

Repeat Parts 2-6 for duration of music.

INSTRUCTIONS:

Ready position is when ball is lying on floor between partners. Do not do part one after first complete sequence.

51

SOCCER

SKILLS: Dribbling

MUSIC: "When The Tough Get Going"

EQUIPMENT: One ball per person in a scattered formation.

PARTS	BEATS	MOVEMENT	DESCRIPTION
1	12	Toe touches.	Two beats per touch. Touch top of ball with toes, alternating right and left feet.
	32	Toe touches.	Same as above except one touch per beat.
	48	Instep dribble.	Close dribble in personal space – one dribble per beat.
	16	Toe touches.	One touch to top of ball per beat, alternating right and left feet.
2	32	Instep dribble.	Close dribble in personal space – one dribble per beat.
	16	Toe touches.	One touch to top of ball per beat, alternating right and left feet.
3	32	Same as Part 2.	Same as Part 2.
	36	Same as Part 2.	Same as Part 2.
	32	Same as Part 2.	Same as Part 2.
	16	Same as Part 2.	Same as Part 2.
	32	Same as Part 2.	Same as Part 2.
	36	Same as Part 2.	Same as Part 2.
	32	Same as Part 2.	Same as Part 2.
	32	Same as Part 2.	Same as Part 2.

PARTS	BEATS	MOVEMENT	DESCRIPTION
4	8	Trunk twists.	Four, two count twists.
	32	Instep dribble.	Close dribble in personal space, one dribble per beat.
	48	Toe touches.	One touch to top of ball per beat, alternating right and left feet.

INSTRUCTIONS:

Each verse is soccer dribbling, each chorus is toe touches. Chorus starts either "When The Going Gets Tough" or "Darling, I'll Climb Any Mountain".

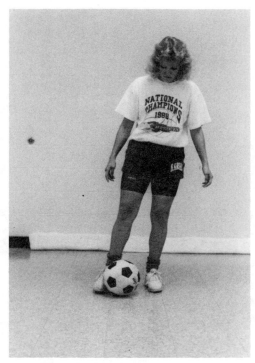

Dribbling In Place

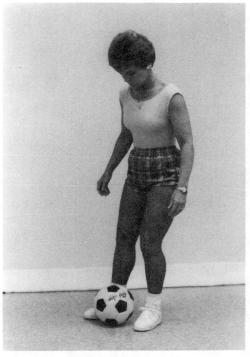

Dribbling While Moving

SOCCER

SKILLS: Dribbling, Kicking, Throw-Ins

MUSIC: "Foot Loose"

EQUIPMENT: None

PARTS	BEATS	MOVEMENT	DESCRIPTION
1	8	Dribble.	Forward
	8	Run.	Backwards
	4	Jog/Kick.	Jog in place three beats. Stationary kick, right foot.
2	4	Jog/Kick.	Jog in place three beats. Stationary kick, left foot.
3	4	Pivot/Throw-in.	Pivot three beats. Overhead throw on last beat.

Repeat the routine until end of music.

INSTRUCTIONS:

It would be helpful to double tape the music or play it twice in order to get the desired time for exercise. Imagery is suggested instead of equipment. However, as skill level improves soccer balls could be used.

SOCCER

SKILLS: Trapping and Kicking

MUSIC: "Don't Stop Till You Get Enough"

EQUIPMENT: None

PARTS	BEATS	MOVEMENT	DESCRIPTION
1	16	Jog.	Slow run.
2	16	Trap.	Trap with left leg, then trap with right. Continue for 16 counts.
3	16	Jog.	Slow run.
4	8	Trap.	Trap with both legs towards the left, then the right.
5	8	Jump and kick.	Jump on left foot kick with right. Jump on right kick with left.

Repeat the routine until end of music.

INSTRUCTIONS:

The number of movements for each part may be determined by the instructor or participant. For example, in Part 2 eight traps (2 per beat) or 16 traps (1 per beat) would be possible. This would depend greatly on an individual's skill level. Imagery is recommended when first starting this routine. As skill levels advance, then soccer balls could be used.

SOCCER

SKILLS: Kicking

MUSIC: "Hyperactive" (Robert Palmer)

EQUIPMENT: Soccer ball for each student.

PARTS	BEATS	MOVEMENT	DESCRIPTION
1	16	Jog.	Slow run.
2	32	In-step kicks.	Move in a square, three steps - then kick - alternating feet.
3	32	Front kicks.	Same as above - switch to shoe lace kicks.
4	24	Front touches.	One foot on top of ball, other on ground, switch to beat.

Repeat the routine until end of music.

INSTRUCTIONS:

The number of movements for each part may vary depending on skill level. It is more important to listen for the beat and move with it, than to be concerned about an exact number of movements per part.

SOCCER

SKILLS: Heading and Kicking

MUSIC: "Would I Lie To You" (The Eurythmics)

EQUIPMENT: None

PARTS	BEATS	MOVEMENT	DESCRIPTION
1	16	Running.	Movement made in a personal space.
	16	Jump-headers.	Three steps, jump, header to left side, then turn body to left side and continue with four counts to each side, 1/4 turn left each time.
2	16	Running.	Movement made in a personal space.
	16	Instep kicks.	Three steps forwards, kick, 1/4 turn left and continue with first step on previous kicking foot using four counts to each side.
3	16	Running.	Movement made in a personal space.
	16	Jump headers.	Same as first time with 1/4 turns to right side.
4	16	Running.	Movement made in a personal space.
	16	Instep kicks.	Same as first time with 1/4 turns to right side.

Repeat the routine until end of music.

INSTRUCTIONS:

Since equipment is not needed, use the technique of imagery as the movements are executed. It is necessary to double tape the music or at least repeat it in order to the desired time.

SOCCER

SKILLS: Dribbling and Throw-Ins

MUSIC: "Can't Stop Til You Get Enough"

EQUIPMENT: None

PARTS	BEATS	MOVEMENT	DESCRIPTION
1	16	Run.	In place or small area.
2	16	Jump.	Around the ball, two beats per jump, make a total of eight jumps.
3	8	Slide shuffle.	More to the right.
	8	Slide shuffle.	Move to the left.
4	16	Overhead throws.	Two beats per throw. Make a total of eight.

Repeat the routine until end of music.

INSTRUCTIONS:

The technique of imagery should be used with this routine, since no equipment is recommended. Equipment could be used with the routine depending on skill and fitness level of the participants.

SOCCER

SKILLS: Footwork and Throw-Ins

MUSIC: "Maneater" (Hall and Oates)

EQUIPMENT: Soccer ball for each participant.

PARTS	BEATS	MOVEMENT	DESCRIPTION
1	16	Jog.	While jogging move arms up and down with the beat.
2	16	Toe tap.	Hopping movement, with each beat toe touch the top of a soccer ball, alternate feet with each beat.
3	8	Dribble.	Moving forwards.
	8	Dribble.	Moving backwards.

Repeat Part 3

PARTS	BEATS	MOVEMENT	DESCRIPTION
4	8	Slide right, throw-in.	Slide right on the first and sixth beat. Throw-in motion on the seventh and eighth beat.
	8	Slide left, throw-in.	Slide left on the first and sixth beat. Throw-in motion on the seventh and eighth beat.

Repeat Part 4

Repeat the routine until end of music.

INSTRUCTIONS:

The routine may be done without the use of equipment. Skill and fitness levels are factors in determining whether or not equipment should be used.

SOCCER

SKILLS: Footwork and Throw-Ins

MUSIC: "It's The Same Old Song" (Four Tops)

EQUIPMENT: Enough soccer balls for one-half of the group.

PARTS	BEATS	MOVEMENT	DESCRIPTION
1	16	Jog and top tap.	Partners facing each other. One person starts with the ball, doing the top tap – other person jogs in place.
2	4	Trap to instep pass.	Partner with ball traps the ball to the count of one, two, three and instep pass on the count of four to partner.

Repeat Part 2 four times.

3	4	Slide right/left overhead pass.	Slide-pass the overhead pass to partner on the third and fourth counts. Slide back and repeat same count.

Repeat the routine until end of music.

INSTRUCTIONS:

The music for this routine should be double taped or played twice for the participants to receive full benefit of the exercise.

SOCCER

SKILLS: Kicking and Throwing

MUSIC: "Dance to the Music" (Sly and the Family Stone)

EQUIPMENT: None

PARTS	BEATS	MOVEMENT	DESCRIPTION
1	16	Running and sprinting.	Alternate steps in-place.
2	16	Kicking (instep).	In a square, pivot after each kick, two left, two right for a four count.
3	16	Throwing (overhead).	Continue square movement formation, for four counts.

Repeat the routine until end of music.

INSTRUCTIONS:

Imagery can be used in this routine, since equipment is not required. When imagery is used, stress the importance of visually imagining the skills being executed properly.

SOCCER

SKILLS: Dribbling, Foot Trapping, and Throw-Ins

MUSIC: "Physical" (Olivia Newton John)

EQUIPMENT: One soccer ball per participant.

PARTS	BEATS	MOVEMENT	DESCRIPTION
1	16	Dribbling.	Move anywhere, keep ball close and do sixteen dribbles.
2	16	Foot traps.	Two beats each, alternating feet. Use four beats to pick up the ball. Do a total of four traps.
3	16	Throw-ins.	Four beats each without releasing ball. Do a total of four.

Repeat the routine until end of music.

INSTRUCTIONS:
Any type of ball that is similar in size to a soccer ball can be used in this routine. It is not necessary to limit the type of ball used to a soccer ball.

SOCCER

SKILLS: Ball Touching

MUSIC: "Money for Nothing" (Dire Straits)

EQUIPMENT: None

PARTS	BEATS	MOVEMENT	DESCRIPTION
1	16	Jog.	Using several spaces.
	8	Kicks.	Heels up on kicks.
	8	Kicks.	Heels back on kicks.
	16	Ball touching.	As if ball were there: touch top of ball with alternating feet. One beat per touch.
2	4	Pivot and step.	Make a circle and pretend to make throw-ins.

Repeat Part 2 four times.

Repeat the routine until end of music.

INSTRUCTIONS:

Imagery is recommended instead of equipment. Skill level of the participants may dictate whether to use equipment or imagery. If equipment is used any type of ball similar to a soccer ball will work.

SOCCER

SKILLS: Throw-Ins and Kicking

MUSIC: "Bad Boys"

EQUIPMENT: None

PARTS	BEATS	MOVEMENT	DESCRIPTION
1	8	Run.	Move in any direction.
2	8	Two hand overhead throw in.	Two beats/throw. Total of four throws.
3	8	Run.	Move in any direction.
4	16	Four behind kicks.	Opposite foot kick behind. Balance foot on fourth beat while running.

Repeat the routine until end of music.

INSTRUCTIONS:

Since no equipment is recommended, imagery can be used. Stress the importance of visually analyzing the skills for proper execution. Soccer type balls may be used with the routine.

SOCCER

SKILLS: Footwork

MUSIC: "You Can't Get What You Want"

EQUIPMENT: None

PARTS	BEATS	MOVEMENT	DESCRIPTION
1	6	Jog.	In place.
	6	Toe taps.	One per beat, imagine having a ball.
	6	Pendulum kicks.	One per beat, imagine ball.
	6	Step right, instep left.	One kick/four beats. Step to side, swing right leg angle forward.
2	6	Step left, instep kick.	Step to side, swing left, leg angle forward.
3	6	Step kicks.	Two beats/step kick. Do a total of three.

Repeat the routine until end of music.

INSTRUCTIONS:

Imagery is recommended for this routine. Footwork is very important when participating in a soccer game. This routine is a good way to practice this skill in a somewhat game like situation.

SOCCER

SKILLS: Kicking and Throw-Ins

MUSIC: "1999" (Prince)

EQUIPMENT: Soccer ball for each participant.

PARTS	BEATS	MOVEMENT	DESCRIPTION
1	16	Kicking.	Hold ball in hands and jog in place for three counts. Step on right foot first.
2	16	Jog in place.	Jog in place making throw-in motion with soccer ball.
3	16	Toe touches.	First four counts place soccer ball on ground. Do toe touches on top of ball for 12 counts.
4	16	Jumping.	Jump over ball side to side, two counts on each side of ball.
5	4	Pick up ball.	

Repeat the routine until end of music.

INSTRUCTIONS:

It is advised to double tape the music or play it twice in order for participants to receive the maximum exercise benefits from the routine.

SOCCER

SKILLS: Running and Dribbling

MUSIC: "Headed to the Future"

EQUIPMENT: None

PARTS	BEATS	MOVEMENT	DESCRIPTION
1	8	Running/arm circles.	Run in place doing arm circle, on last beat turn to your right.
	8	Running/arm circles.	Run in place doing arm circle, on last beat turn to your right.
	8	Running/arm circles.	Run in place doing arm circle, on last beat turn to your right.
	8	Running/arm circles.	Run in place doing arm circle, on last beat turn to your right.
2	8	Slide step.	Slide step to your right.
	8	Slide step.	Slide step to your left.
3	8	Dribble.	Dribble forward.
4	8	Run.	Run backwards.

Repeat the routine until music ends.

INSTRUCTIONS:

This is a good routine for participants to learn how to analyze their skills through proper execution without trying to control a soccer ball. This is a good routine for the beginner in soccer and is also adequate as a warm-up for the skilled player.

SOCCER

SKILLS: Kicking

MUSIC: "Stay the Night" (Latoya Jackson)

EQUIPMENT: Soccer ball for each participant

PARTS	BEATS	MOVEMENT	DESCRIPTION
1	16	Jog.	In place or around workout area.
2	32	Instep kicks.	Move in a square, take three steps – then kick alternating feet.
3	32	Front kicks.	Same as above but switch to shoe lace kicks.
4	24	Front touches.	One foot on top of ball, the other on ground, switch to beat.

Repeat the routine until end of music.

INSTRUCTIONS:

Repeat the music for at least two or three times to give the participant the maximum exercise benefits. It is also easy to add new movement to this routine. New movements could intensify the aerobic activity of the routine.

SELECTED BIBLIOGRAPHY

Ford, G. Basic Soccer: Strategies for Successful Player and Program Development. Boston, Mass: Allyn and Bacon, Inc., 1982.

Ford, G. and Kane, J. Go for Goal: Winning Drills and Exercises for Soccer. Newton, MASS: Allyn and Bacon, Inc., 1985.

Gabbard, C., Leblanc, E., and Lowy, S. Physical Education for Children. Englewood Cliffs, N.J.: Prentice Hall, Inc., 1987.

Morris, D., and Stiehl, J. Physical Education: From Intent to Action. Columbus, OH: Charles E. Merrill Publishing Co., 1985.

SKILLS USED IN SOFTBALL ROUTINES

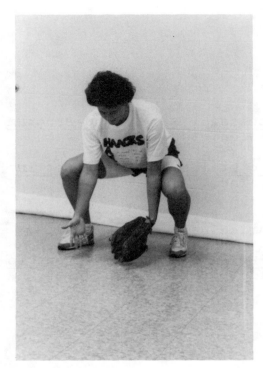

Fielding The Ball

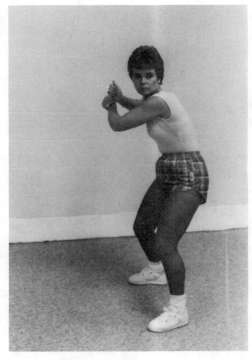

Batting Without Bat

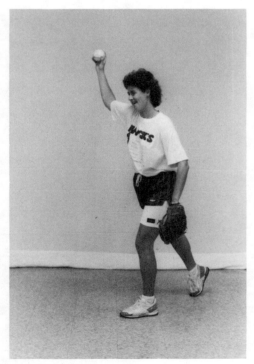

Throwing

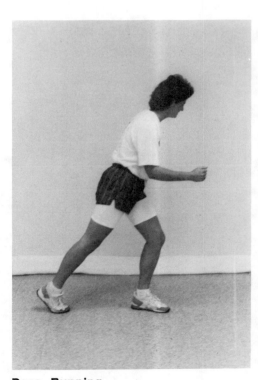

Base Running

CHAPTER 7

SOFTBALL

Softball is a very popular recreational sport. Many people of all ages have found the slow pitch version to be a very exciting and rewarding experience. For those who want to develop and use more advanced skills, the fast pitch version is more likely to meet their needs. The popularity of softball in the United States and in many other countries is probably due to the game's ease and safety. In fact, it is a game where very little protective equipment is required. Regardless of whether an individual is playing in the slow pitch or fast pitch version, there must be proficiency in the skills of throwing, catching, and batting. These skills can only be developed and maintained through personal fitness programs. More specifically the fitness activities should directly relate to the movements required to execute softball skills.

SOFTBALL AND FITNESS

Softball is a game that requires an individual to have many movement skills that do not relate to the skills of throwing, catching, and batting. For example, the game requires running, jumping, stretching, bending, twisting, and turning. As with many other sports, these movements directly relate to physical fitness and cardiovascular endurance.

An individual may participate in the game of softball for many different reasons. Regardless of the reason, all people want to experience success as they play the game. Individual performance depends on overall physical fitness as it relates to the sport of softball. It seems logical to develop a fitness level that directly relates to softball. This simply implies that an individual should practice and develop skills that are game like in nature.

Strength and Endurance

The range of movement in the game of softball varies a great deal. Depending on the nature of any given play, a movement that had never been practiced could be required at any time. Participation in a sport with many movements requires strength and cardiovascular endurance, especially when new and unpracticed movements maybe required.

Upper and lower body strength are equally important to execute softball skills. The skills of throwing and catching a softball require good arm and shoulder strength. Running skills are also very important to the softball player. The legs are used on both offense and defense in situations where speed and agility are required. As a result the strength of the lower body is a necessary characteristic for being an effective softball player.

Strength and endurance for softball participation can be developed and maintained through player exercise. Because softball requires an individual to have a variety of movement skills, a specific type of fitness is required for proper skill execution. The aerobic routines for softball are designed to improve an individual's strength and endurance.

SOFTBALL ROUTINES

There are fourteen aerobic routines designed around softball skills. The routines will help promote aerobic fitness and aid in the development and/or refinement of softball skills. Softball skills used in the development of these routines are listed in Figure 7.1

1.	Fielding	5.	Base Running
2.	Batting	6.	Agility Running
3.	Throwing	7.	Balance
4.	Catching	8.	Tossing

FIGURE 7.1 Basic softball skills for which
the routines are developed.

The skills, movements, and music may be changed or modified for each routine. A music change may require the movements to be choreographed differently. Skill and movement changes must maintain good flow.

These routines can be used for all ages. Skill and fitness levels of the participants should be considered when selecting routines for exercise. Continuous movement is a critical factor for the participants in all routines.

SOFTBALL

SKILLS: Hand Positions for Fielding and Batting

MUSIC: "Nothing at All" (Heart)

EQUIPMENT: None

PARTS	BEATS	MOVEMENT	DESCRIPTION
1	16	Running.	In place.
	16	Shuffle fielding.	Shuffle sideways, scoop with hands low, and repeat to same side, then reverse to other side, two times to each side.
2	16	Running.	In place.
	16	Hitting.	Face dominant side with that hand in fist on top of other hand in fist, use two counts to pull hands behind body, one count step front foot sideways, one count swing, repeat entire motion four times.

Repeat the routine until end of music.

INSTRUCTIONS:

Imagery is recommended instead to using equipment. If participants have above average skill level in softball, then equipment can be used.

SOFTBALL

SKILLS: Throwing and Catching

MUSIC: "Do Not Disturb"

EQUIPMENT: None

PARTS	BEATS	MOVEMENT	DESCRIPTION
1	32	Sliding.	Slide side to side, eight counts to each side. Keep hands low between straddled legs.
2	32	Throwing.	Sixteen throws alternating arms. Jump back on one, throw on four, four counts for each throw.
3	32	Fielding.	Run forward three counts, catch ball on fourth count. Run backwards three counts, catch ball on fourth count.

Repeat the routine until end of music.

INSTRUCTIONS:

Encourage participants to keep the rear tucked under when fielding the grounders. Imagery is suggested unless the participants have an above average skill level.

SOFTBALL

SKILLS: Fielding and Throwing

MUSIC: "What Have You Got For Me Lately" (Janet Jackson)

EQUIPMENT: One softball or equivalent per two students.

PARTS	BEATS	MOVEMENT	DESCRIPTION
1	32	Jog.	In place or in a small area.
2	8	Fielding and throwing.	Slide three counts to right, field on five and throw on seven.
		Rolling and catching.	Slide three counts to left, roll on fourth and catch on the eighth count.
		(Do this two times.)	
	8	Running.	Change position with partner and change roles.
	8	Rolling and catching.	Slide three counts to left, roll on fourth and catch on the eighth count.
		Partner field and throw.	Slide three counts to right, field on the fifth and throw on the seventh count.
		(Do this two times.)	
	8	Running.	Change positions with partner and change roles.

Repeat the routine until end of music.

INSTRUCTIONS:

Any type of ball that is similar to the size of a softball can be used. Skill level of participants should be considered when selecting balls to use.

SOFTBALL

SKILLS: Batting Swing

MUSIC: "California Girls" (David Lee Roth)

EQUIPMENT: None

PARTS	BEATS	MOVEMENT	DESCRIPTION
1	16	Jumping Jacks.	Two to the right, two to the left.
2	8	Slides.	Four to the right, our back.
3	16	Jog.	Jog while swinging arms to front.
4	4	Bat swings.	Swing bat four times.

Repeat the routine until end of music.

INSTRUCTIONS:

In Part 4 imagery is recommended due to safety. If doing the routine in a large open space then bats could be scattered around the area to use in this routine. Skill level of the participants would also be a factor.

SOFTBALL

SKILLS: Tossing and Catching

MUSIC: "Theme From the Greatest American Hero"

EQUIPMENT: One softball per circle of 10-12.

PARTS	BEATS	MOVEMENT	DESCRIPTION
1	60	Sliding, tossing, catching.	Students slide counter-clockwise around circle. Student with the ball will toss it across the circle to someone who catches it and tosses it to someone else.
	96	Sliding, tossing, catching.	Circle changes to clockwise direction while continuing to toss the ball.
2	84	Same as Part 1.	Circle changes to counter-clockwise direction.
	40	Same as Part 1.	Circle changes to clockwise direction.
	40	Same as Part 1.	Circle changes to counter-clockwise direction.
3	80	Same as Part 2.	Circle changes to clockwise direction.

INSTRUCTIONS:

Circle changes directions on chorus -- "Believe It or Not." Underarm or sidearm tossing motion may be used. Routine is for average or above skill level.

SOFTBALL

SKILLS: Running the Bases and Batting

MUSIC: "Walk of Life"

EQUIPMENT: Four softball bases or equivalent.

PARTS	BEATS	MOVEMENT	DESCRIPTION
1	80	Running bases.	Four steps per beat.
	16*	Batting movements.	Four counts each. Step forward—step, together equal two counts. Step backward—step together equal two counts. Batting arm movements on two counts.
2	48	Running bases.	Same as in Part 1.
	32*	Fielding positions.	Four count deep knee bends. Hands touch the ground as if fielding the ball.
3	144	Running bases.	Same as in Part 2.

* There are two short instrumental sections between the verses.

INSTRUCTIONS:

Imagery is recommended for the batting movements. To receive aerobic exercise benefit, double tape the music or repeat it. The routine should be done at least two times.

SOFTBALL

SKILLS: Fielding and Throwing

MUSIC: "Wanna Be Starting Something" (Michael Jackson)

EQUIPMENT: None

PARTS	BEATS	MOVEMENT	DESCRIPTION
1	16	Running.	In place.
	16	Field ground ball (4).	Four beats per up/down motion to field ball.
2	8	Running.	To the right.
	8	Running.	To the left.
	16	Throwing.	Four beats per throw. Total of four throws.
3	8	Running.	To the right.
	8	Running.	To the left.

Repeat the routine until end of music.

INSTRUCTIONS:
Imagery is recommended for this routine. Balls and gloves may be used, if participants are of average or above average skill.

SOFTBALL

SKILLS: Fielding and Catching

MUSIC: "Nine to Five" (Dolly Parton)

EQUIPMENT: Softball gloves.

PARTS	BEATS	MOVEMENT	DESCRIPTION
1	8	Jogging.	In place or around area.
	8	Fielding grounders.	Jog to the right eight counts, continue turning right until you complete a square. On the seventh and eighth beat bend for a ground ball, turn right on the first beat and repeat.
2	8	Slide right.	Tag base with right toe on the eighth beat.
	8	Slide left.	Tag base with left toe on the eighth beat.

(Repeat Part 2 four times.)

| 3 | 8 | Jumping. | Jump high, with hands high over head to catch a high fly ball. |

Repeat the routine until music ends.

INSTRUCTIONS:

Imagery is recommended for fielding ground balls and catching fly balls. Participants can still use gloves during imagery.

SOFTBALL

SKILLS: Fielding and Catching

MUSIC: Axel F" (Soundtrack Beverly Hills Cop)

EQUIPMENT: One softball per participant.

PARTS	BEATS	MOVEMENT	DESCRIPTION
1	16	Lunges.	Two count lunges from side to side rolling softball from one hand to the other across the floor.
	16	Jogging.	One jog and toss per beat. Jog in place tossing ball from one hand to the other.
2	16	Bend knees and lower body.	Two counts down to bend and lower body. Two counts up. Repeat four times forming square.
	16	Jogging.	Four counts per toss. Toss ball five feet in air and catch with two hands while jogging.
3	32	Toss ball and sprinting.	Eight counts to complete. Toss ball ahead six to eight feet, spring forward to get in front of ball and field it. Repeat four times going in any direction.

Repeat the routine until music ends.

INSTRUCTIONS:

This routine is designed for participants who have average to above average skill levels.

SOFTBALL

SKILLS: Fielding and Throwing

MUSIC: "Nothing At All" (Heart)

EQUIPMENT: None

PARTS	BEATS	MOVEMENT	DESCRIPTION
1	16	Running and sprinting.	Alternate running and sprinting in place.
	16	Shuffling and fielding.	Shuffle side to side, lower both hands on third beat, field and bring up hands on fourth beat. Four count, repeat twice.
	4	Shuffle steps.	In place catch-up. Participant should try to get back on beat, if off.
2	16	Fielding and throwing.	Four count, keep head down on the fielding, square up and throw on the fourth beat. Do a 1/3 turn swing on each throw, alternating left to right.

Repeat the routine until music ends.

INSTRUCTIONS:

Imagery is recommended for the fielding and throwing parts of this routine. If participants are above average in skill level, then equipment could be used.

SOFTBALL

SKILLS: Batting, Fielding and Throwing

MUSIC: "Happy days"

EQUIPMENT: Four softball bases or equivalent.

PARTS	BEATS	MOVEMENT	DESCRIPTION
1	12	Batting.	Make three batting swings. Four beats per swing.
2	16	Running.	Follow the bases using four beats between each base.
3	8	Sliding.	To the right.
4	8	Fielding and throwing.	One time only. Four beats to field and four to throw.
5	8	Slides.	To the left.
6	8	Fielding and throwing.	One time only. Four beats to field and four to throw.
7	16	Run.	Follow the bases using four beats between each base.

Repeat the routine until end of music.

INSTRUCTIONS:

Imagery is recommended for batting, fielding and throwing. If participants have above average skill level, then equipment may be used.

SOFTBALL

SKILLS: Batting Swing

MUSIC: "The Heat Is On" (Glenn Fry)

EQUIPMENT: None

PARTS	BEATS	MOVEMENT	DESCRIPTION
1	8	Bat swings.	Two beats per swing. Do four swings.
	16	Jogging.	In place.
2	8	Bat swings.	Two beats per swing. Do four swings.
	16	Jogging.	In place while circling arms forward.
3	8	Bat swings.	Two beats per swing. Do four swings.
	16	Jogging.	In place while crossing arms at shoulder height.
4	8	Bat swings.	Two beats per swing. Do four swings.
	16	Jogging.	In place while circling arms backward.

Repeat the routine until end of music.

INSTRUCTIONS:

Imagery is recommended for the bat swinging. If skill level of participants is above average softball balls can be used. Doubling taping of the music is suggested in order to make the routine more aerobic.

SOFTBALL

SKILLS: Fielding and Throwing

MUSIC: "Wanna Be Startin Something" (Michael Jackson)

EQUIPMENT: None

PARTS	BEATS	MOVEMENT	DESCRIPTION
1	8	Fielding.	Bend at waist, scoop up ball. Do this four times.
	8	Fielding and throwing.	Bend at waist, scoop up ball and throw it. Do this two times.
2	8	Jogging.	Moving to the right or left.
	8	Fielding and throwing.	Same as in Part 1.
3	8	Jogging.	Moving right or left. Keep low to floor.

Repeat the routine until end of music.

INSTRUCTIONS:

Imagery is recommended for the fielding and throwing movements. If participants were above average in skills, the routine could easily be modified to use a softball and a softball glove.

SOFTBALL

SKILLS: Batting, Catching, Fielding, Throwing and Base Running

MUSIC: "Sisters Are Doing It For Themselves"

EQUIPMENT: Softball Bases or Equivalent.

PARTS	BEATS	MOVEMENT	DESCRIPTION
1	16	Batting.	Make warm-up swing, two beats per swing. Do this four times. Make homerun swing, two beats per swing. Do this four times.
2	8	Jogging forward.	Catch pop fly on eighth beat.
	8	Jogging backward.	Catch pop fly on eighth beat.
3	16	Sliding steps-right.	Four beats to slide, two beats to field, two beats to throw. Do this two times.
4	48	Base running.	Use twelve beats per base, making 1/4 turn to the left on each base. Do this four times or for four bases.
5	128	Repeat Parts 2 and 3 two times.	
6	48	Base running.	Use twelve beats per base, making 1/4 turn to the left on each base. Do this four times or for four bases.
	16	Pitching and catching.	Use two beats to pitch and two beats to catch. Do this four times.
7	16	Repeat Part 1.	

Repeat the routine until end of music.

INSTRUCTIONS:

Imagery is recommended but softballs and gloves may be used depending on the skill level of the routine. This routine is designed for those participants that have established a good level of cardiovascular fitness and have at least average softball skills.

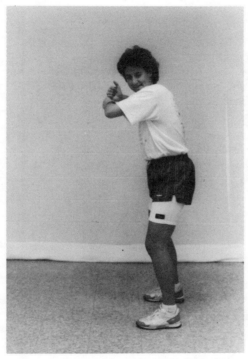

Using Imagery To Practice Batting

SELECTED BIBLIOGRAPHY

Drysdale, S. and Harris, K. Complete Handbook of Winning Softball. Boston, MASS: Allyn and Bacon, Inc., 1982.

Nichols, B. Moving and Learning: The Elementary School Physical Education Experience. St. Louis, MO: Times Mirror/Mosby College Publishing, 1986.

Morris, D. and Stiehl, J. Physical Education: From Intent to Action. Columbus, OH: Charles E. Merrill Publishing Co., 1985.

SKILLS USED IN TOUCH FOOTBALL ROUTINES

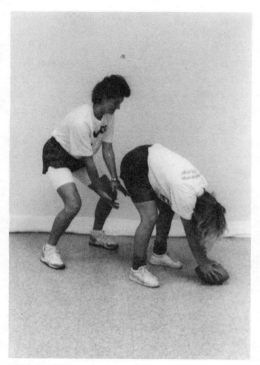

Hiking With A Partner

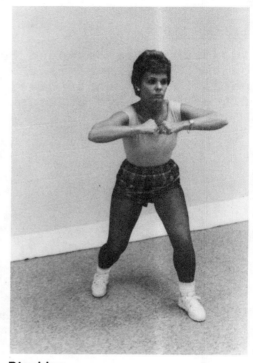

Blocking

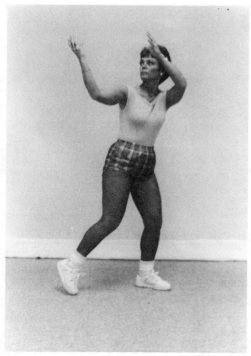

Catching The Ball

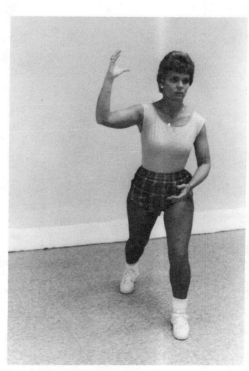

Throwing Without Ball

CHAPTER 8

TOUCH FOOTBALL

Touch football games are excellent activities for promoting physical fitness. The games require a variety of movement skills. Unfortunately, many people participate in these games on an irregular basis. Usually, touch football is played as a pick-up holiday type of game. It seems to be somewhat of a revitalized sport activity in public school .physical education curriculums at both the elementary and secondary levels. If public school students become more skilled in the game of touch football, it may become a popular recreational sport of the future. More people may recognize this sport as a good form of physical exercise.

TOUCH FOOTBALL AND FITNESS

Many individuals who participate in touch football games fail to recognize that it is much like any other sport. To successfully participate in the game, a certain level of cardiovascular fitness is required. Without this type of fitness, it is difficult to execute the skills properly for a period of time. When there is a good level of cardiovascular fitness, an individual can play the game of touch football the way it should be played. When played properly, touch football can tax the cardiovascular system of the participants, therefore it is a good form of exercise and physical activity.

Touch Football Skills

Skills needed to participate in touch football are refined versions of basic motor skills. The game requires a lot of running (sprinting and short distance), agility movement, catching, throwing, passings, eye hand and eye foot skills. Practicing these skills in a game like or continuous movement experience enables the individual to develop or improve their fitness level that is sport specific.

Strength and Endurance

For the previously mentioned skills to be developed, a specific level of strength and endurance is necessary. Like any other sport, touch football is a game where strength and endurance enhances the chances for successful participation. In this particular sport total body strength is important, if the participant is to experience success. Endurance is also critical because most people who play the game want to participate on a continuous basis for one to three hours.

The endurance factor can determine whether or not an individual participates in a safe and healthy manner. With increased strength and endurance, individuals can participate in the sport of touch football on a consistent and regular basis.

TOUCH FOOTBALL ROUTINES

The following aerobic routines were developed to improve cardiovascular fitness and enhance the development or improvement of motor skills necessary for participation in the sport of touch football. The fourteen routines can easily be modified or changed to meet the skill and fitness levels of the participants.

The routines for touch football were developed using the skills listed in Figure 8.1.

1.	Blocking	6.	Catching
2.	Agility	7.	Pitching
3.	Passing	8.	Kicking
4.	Hiking	9.	Running
5.	Handing-Off	10.	Tagging/Touching

FIGURE 8.1 Basic touch football skills for
which the routines were developed.

Music other than that recommended may be used. A music change may require the movements be choreographed differently than that described. When changes are made, it is important to keep a good flow to the movements.

The routines are recommended to be used with ages ten and up. Skill and fitness levels of the participants should be considered in determining what routine(s) are to be used with a particular group. Regardless of the routine, continuous movement must always be encouraged.

TOUCH FOOTBALL

SKILLS: Blocking and Dodging

MUSIC: "California Girls" (Beach Boys)

EQUIPMENT: None

PARTS	BEATS	MOVEMENT	DESCRIPTION
1	8	Run.	To find a person and face them.
	4	Jog/Clap.	Jog in place/clap on last beat.
2	8	Dodging.	Side to side four times shifting weight. Right to left foot, etc.
3	4	Blocking.	Hands up no contact.
	8	Run.	To find a new person.

Repeat the routine until end of music.

INSTRUCTIONS:

For safety of the participants, the technique of imagery is recommended. The skill level of the participants may help the leader determine whether or not to use this technique.

TOUCH FOOTBALL

SKILLS: Passing and Faking

MUSIC: "Do You Believe in Love" (Huey Lewis and the News)

EQUIPMENT: None

PARTS	BEATS	MOVEMENT	DESCRIPTION
1	16	Forward/backward running.	Four steps forward, four steps backward, two times each way.
	16	Passing.	Two counts to cock ball, one count each to step and throw. Repeat four times.
2	16	Forward/backward running.	Four steps forward, four steps backward, two times each way.
	16	Faking.	Long step and lean body sideways, repeat to the other side, eight times to each side.

Repeat the routine until end of music.

INSTRUCTIONS:

Imagery is recommended for the passing and faking movements. If the skill level of the participants is above average, footballs may be used for these movements.

TOUCH FOOTBALL

SKILLS: Holding the Football

MUSIC: "Glory Days" (Bruce Springsteen)

EQUIPMENT: Football for each person.

PARTS	BEATS	MOVEMENT	DESCRIPTION
1	16	Side to side jumps.	Feet together holding ball.
	16	Eight leg kicks.	Two beats per kick, kick toward extended football.
2	16	Side to side jumps.	Feet together holding ball.
	16	Eight leg kicks.	Two beats per kick, kick toward extended football.

(Continue holding the ball in hands for the duration of routine.)

PARTS	BEATS	MOVEMENT	DESCRIPTION
3	2	Stretch movements on each bounce.	Bounce forward two beats.
	2	Stretch movements on each bounce.	Bounce right two beats.
	2	Stretch movements on each bounce.	Bounce back two beats.
	2	Stretch movements on each bounce.	Bounce left two beats.

Repeat the routine until end of music.

TOUCH FOOTBALL

SKILLS: Catching and Throwing

MUSIC: "Don't Stop 'till You Get Enough" (Michael Jackson)

EQUIPMENT: One football for every two participants.

PARTS	BEATS	MOVEMENT	DESCRIPTION
1	32	Jog.	Jog in place or around area.
2	16	Jog and throw.	Jog for four beats, then participants with footballs throw to ones without the balls on the seventh beat. Repeat on next eight beats.
	16	Jog and throw.	Same as above.
	8	Jog and rotate.	Every one proceeds to next point on square (counter-clockwise direction). During rotation, person moving to #3 spot toss ball across to person moving to #1 spot.
3	16	Jog and throw.	Jog for four beats, then participants with footballs throw to ones without the balls on the seventh beat. Repeat for next eight beats.
	16	Jog and throw.	Same as above.
	8	Jog and rotate.	Same as in Part 2.

Repeat Parts 2 and 3 until end of music.

INSTRUCTIONS:

To start this routine, it is recommended to have groups of four stand on four points of a square, numbered counter-clockwise 1-2-3-4. Participants on spots one and two start with the footballs.

TOUCH FOOTBALL

SKILLS: Holding the Football

MUSIC: "Wanna Be Startin' Something" (Michael Jackson)

EQUIPMENT: One football per participant.

PARTS	BEATS	MOVEMENT	DESCRIPTION
1	16	Jog.	Jog in the circle holding football running in clockwise direction.
	16	Jog.	Same as above except run counter clockwise.
2	16	Twists.	Twist body to the right while holding ball in front, then twist to the left. Use eight beats per direction.
3	16	Pass.	One participant drops the football. The others in group begin passing all the footballs in clockwise direction.

Repeat the routine until end of music.

INSTRUCTIONS:

All participants form a circle, after each has a football. Imagery can be used, should the leader decide not to use footballs. Should enough footballs not be available, participants without footballs can use imagery.

TOUCH FOOTBALL

SKILLS: Pitching and Catching

MUSIC: "Bobby Sue" (Oak Ridge Boys)

EQUIPMENT: One football per two concentric circles.

PARTS	BEATS	MOVEMENT	DESCRIPTION
1	84	Jogging/pitching/ catching.	One circle jogging clockwise and one circle jogging counter-clockwise. Use one step per beat. Student with football will pitch ball to someone coming toward them in the other circle who catches it and does likewise.
2	128	Jogging/pitching/ catching.	Circles change directions. Movement same as in Part 1.
	96	Jogging/pitching/ catching.	Circles change directions. Movement same as in Part 1.
	32	Jogging/pitching/ catching.	Circles change directions. Movement same as in Part 1.
	32	Jogging/pitching/ catching.	Circles change directions. Movement same as in Part 1.

Repeat the routine until end of music.

INSTRUCTIONS:

Circles are to change directions every time "B,B,B,Bobby Sue" is played. If participants have trouble counting beats, routine can easily be changed so movements are to a lower number of beats.

TOUCH FOOTBALL

SKILLS: Hiking and Kicking

MUSIC: "Wanna Be Startin Something" (Michael Jackson)

EQUIPMENT: None

PARTS	BEATS	MOVEMENT	DESCRIPTION
1	8	Slide shuffle right.	Clap on beats four and eight.
	8	Slide shuffle left.	Clap on beats four and eight.
2	16	Hike.	Four beats per hike/ straighten body position.
3	12	Run.	In place.
	4	Hop.	In place.
4	1	Kick.	
	7	Run.	In place.

Do Part 4 four times before starting the routine over.
Repeat the routine until end of music.

INSTRUCTIONS:
Imagery is recommended, however, if skill level of participants is average or above average footballs could be used.

TOUCH FOOTBALL

SKILLS: Catching, Faking and Running Pass Patterns.

MUSIC: "It's The Same Old Song" (The Four Tops)

EQUIPMENT: None

PARTS	BEATS	MOVEMENT	DESCRIPTION
1	16	Running.	In place four counts, forward and backwards two times.
2	16	Catching and faking.	In place, four counts, alternate side tuck and fake. Catch-tuck-fake-go is the sequence to follow.
3	4	Running.	Catch up with beat, if behind. If not continue running with beat.
4	32	Running pass patterns.	First time cut on fourth count, give a fake on your cut. Second time through, cut on the eighth count. Continue same pattern for 32 counts.

Repeat the routine until end of music.

INSTRUCTIONS:

Imagery is recommended for this routine. The movements have to be quick and the participants must demonstrate quick reflexive action in order to stay with the beat.

TOUCH FOOTBALL

SKILLS: Tagging, Hiking, Holding the Ball

MUSIC: "Eye of the Tiger"

EQUIPMENT: One football per two participants.

PARTS	BEATS	MOVEMENT	DESCRIPTION
1	16	Run and tag.	Number one holds the ball correctly and runs.
			Number two tries to touch number one with two hands on the back tag.
2	12	Hiking.	Number one hikes ball to number two, both turn around.
			Number two hikes ball to number one, both turn around.
3	16	Run and tag.	Number one tries to tag number two.
			Number two hikes to number one, both turn.
4	12	Hikes.	Number two hikes to number two, both turn.
			Number two hikes to number one.

Repeat the routine until end of music.

INSTRUCTIONS:

This routine is designed for those of average or above average skills in touch football. If skill levels are below average, the technique of imagery can be used. Participants start the routine in sets of twos.

TOUCH FOOTBALL

SKILLS: Passing and Hiking

MUSIC: "You Wear It Well"

EQUIPMENT: None

PARTS	BEATS	MOVEMENT	DESCRIPTION
1	8	Pass.	Four beats per pass.
	8	Jogging.	Move to the right.
2	8	Hiking.	Four beats per hike.
	8	Jogging.	Move to the left.

Repeat the routine until end of music.

INSTRUCTIONS:

The technique of imagery is recommended. If skill levels of participants is average, footballs may be used.

TOUCH FOOTBALL

SKILLS: Passing and Catching

MUSIC: "Oh Jungleland"

EQUIPMENT: One football per every two participants.

PARTS	BEATS	MOVEMENT	DESCRIPTION
1	32	Scissors kicks.	Forward on one beat, backward on one beat.
2	8	Jogging.	One beat per step, circle right.
3	16	Passing and receiving.	To a partner, use four beats to pass, four beats to receive. Jog in place while passing and receiving.
4	8	Jogging.	To find a new partner.

Repeat the routine until end of music.

INSTRUCTIONS:

If participants have difficulty with the routine, use imagery instead of the footballs. Skill level can dictate which technique is appropriate.

TOUCH FOOTBALL

SKILLS: Defensive Moves, Passing, Catching, and Blocking

MUSIC: "Theme From Peter Gunn"

EQUIPMENT: None

PARTS	BEATS	MOVEMENT	DESCRIPTION
1	32	Defensive shuffle.	Circling to right for sixteen beats, to the left for sixteen beats.
2	32	Defensive back jogging.	Go forward sixteen beats, backward sixteen beats.
	16	Fade backward and throw forward.	Take fading steps backward for three beats and throw on fourth beat. Do this a total of four times.
3	32	Jogging.	To the right and catch pass on eighth beat. Then, to the right and catch pass on eighth beat. Do two times.
	8	Jogging.	Moving to the right, knock down pass on seventh and eighth beats.
	8	Sprinting.	Moving backwards intercept pass on seventh and eighth beats.
	8	Jogging.	Moving to the left, knock down pass on seventh and eighth beats.
	8	Sprinting.	Moving backwards intercept pass on seventh and eighth beats.
4	32	Sliding steps.	Moving to the right, try to throw pass in a pass blocking situation. Throw on seventh and eighth beats but keep the ball. Repeat moving to the left. Use a total of sixteen beats. Repeat these movements.

PARTS	BEATS	MOVEMENT	DESCRIPTION
5	80	Running pass patterns.	Run individual pass patterns. Use eight beats per patterns. Example of pattern is: jog forward six beats, head fake left on the seventh beat, but go right on eighth beat. Important to improvise own pass patterns.

Repeat the routine until end of music.

INSTRUCTIONS:

Imagery is recommended for this routine. It is a good exercise for the participants to develop the ability to analyze their own movements and develop creative passing options.

TOUCH FOOTBALL

SKILLS: Kicking and Catching

MUSIC: "Dancing in the Streets"

EQUIPMENT: One football for each participant.

PARTS	BEATS	MOVEMENT	DESCRIPTION
1	16	Jog.	Jog in place with football tucked.
2	16	Four catches and tucks.	Two counts per catch and two counts per tuck. Continue to jog in place as moves are executed.
3	16	Eight kicks.	Extend arms in front with ball in hands. Kick leg up to ball, left leg first. Two counts for each kick.

Repeat the routine until end of music.

TOUCH FOOTBALL

SKILLS: Slide Stepping and Defensive Movements

MUSIC: "Wanna Be Startin' Something" (Michael Jackson)

EQUIPMENT: None

PARTS	BEATS	MOVEMENT	DESCRIPTION
1	32	Jogging.	Fast jogging facing a partner about three to four feet apart.
2	16	Slide steps.	Sliding movements to the right, partners split. Use eight beats. Repeat the movement to the left.

Do Part 2 two times.

PARTS	BEATS	MOVEMENT	DESCRIPTION
3	32	Jogging.	Same as in Part 1.

Repeat the routine until end of music.

SELECTED BIBLIOGRAPHY

Moore, D., Misher, F.F., Rink, J.E. Sports and Recreational Activities for Men and Women. 9th ed. St. Louis, MO: Times Mirror/Mosby College Publishing, 1987.

Pangrazi, R.P. and Darst, P.W. Dynamic Physical Education Curriculum and Instruction. Minneapolis, MN: Burgess Publishing Company, 1985.

Singer, R.N. Coaching, Athletics, and Psychology. New York, NY: McGraw-Hill Book Company, 1972.

SKILLS USED IN VOLLEYBALL ROUTINES

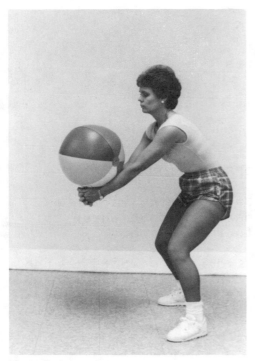

Bumping

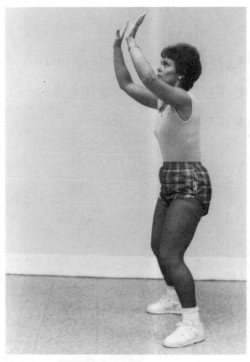

Setting Without Ball

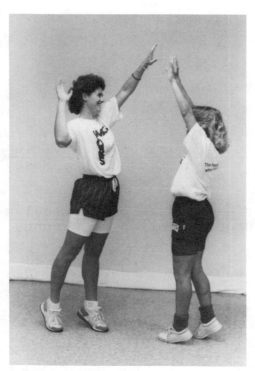

Spiking and Blocking

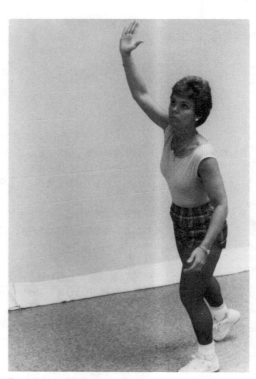

Serving Without Ball

CHAPTER 9

VOLLEYBALL

Volleyball is a game played by millions of people. The popularity of the game is probably due to the game's simplicity and contribution to physical fitness. Society's increased interest in fitness activities has more than likely been a contributing factor to the increased participation in the sport of volleyball. For many people the game of volleyball has become an alternative to traditional fitness activities. The increased interest in volleyball has also been due to the fact that it is a fun and enjoyable game to play. When people have fun in a fitness related experience, it usually becomes one that is repeated on a regular basis. Volleyball has become more popular in elementary, junior high, and high school physical education programs which means the carryover value of it into adulthood is more likely to happen. As a result, the need to develop and maintain good skill and fitness level certainly exists.

VOLLEYBALL AND FITNESS

All sport related games requires certain skills. Volleyball is no exception. All sports require the participants to have a certain level of fitness. Volleyball is no exception. Some volleyball skills are very difficult to execute. Most of the skills can be modified or have some degree of variation in skill execution. This does make it easier for individuals to participate and enjoy the game. Basically, people who want to play volleyball must be aerobically and physically fit. A good level of fitness can aid in the development and main- tenance of volleyball skills. Success in skill execution can be a self motivator for generating an individual's interest to play volleyball on a regular basis.

Volleyball Skills

There are two basic skills in volleyball. These are serving and volleying the ball. An individual must be able to execute these skills before playing the game. These skills actually initiate the movement in the game. Without the skills, the benefits of exercise would be somewhat limited. There are other skills in volleyball to be learned but serving and volleying must come first.

There is one distinct advantage in the development of volleyball skills. The advantage is in the fact that there is more than one way to perform most of the skills. For example, there are two or three different and acceptable ways to serve the ball. This increases an individual's chances of finding a way to successfully and consistently serve the volleyball. The long term effect of variations is skill execution is that more people are likely to participate in volleyball for exercise.

Strength and Endurance

Once the action starts in a game of volleyball, the movements and skills required vary greatly. Many times participants in the game have to recall previously learned motor skills that are indirectly related to game. If the participants have good upper and lower body strength, the chances of proper skill execution are greater. A good example of the need for upper body strength is in the skill of serving. One must have enough arm and shoulder strength to hit the ball hard enough on the serve for the ball to go on to the opponents court. Strength can also affect the control of the hit. An example of lower body strength is the amount of jumping required in volleyball. Good leg strength is important because several volleyball skills require a jump before the actual skill can be executed.

As with most sports, volleyball is no different when it comes to the endurance factor. When participants have a good cardiovascular fitness level their ability to properly execute skills in game-like situations is certainly enhanced. Developing and maintaining cardiovascular fitness will also allow individuals to participate in a game of volleyball for a longer period of time without skill execution being negatively affected. Like other sports, volleyball is unique in that the fitness required for successful participation is specific to the sport. One can overall be physically fit, but would need to achieve a fitness level appropriate for the game of volleyball. Sport specific aerobic routines can help develop this type of fitness.

VOLLEYBALL ROUTINES

The following sport specific aerobic routines were developed to improve cardiovascular fitness and enhance the development or improvement of skills needed to participate in the game of volleyball. The fifteen routines can be modified or changed to meet the skill or fitness levels of the participants.

The routines for volleyball were developed using the skills listed in Figure 9.1.

1.	Volleying	4.	Serving
2.	Bumping	5.	Passing
3.	Setting	6.	Blocking

FIGURE 9.1   Basic volleyball skills for which the routines were developed.

If the movements in these routines are changed, it maybe necessary to change music in order for the flow to be good. On the other hand, a music change may require a skill or movement adjustment. Some of the volleyball routines were developed for aiding in the learning of positions and rotation. When first developing skills for volleyball, this alone can be a challenging experience.

The routines are recommended for ages twelve and up. Skill and fitness levels of the participants should be considered when determining what routines should be used with a particular group. For all of the routines, continuous movement must be encouraged at all times.

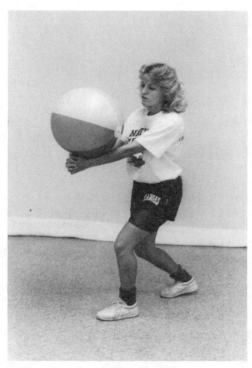

Using Beachball To Bump

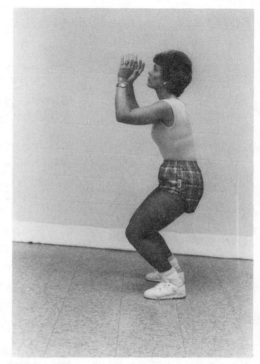

Using Imagery To Develop Skills

VOLLEYBALL

SKILLS: Volleying

MUSIC: "Physical" (Olivia Newton-John)

EQUIPMENT: Beachballs (1-3 per group of 20 or less)

PARTS	BEATS	MOVEMENT	DESCRIPTION
1	16	Short jumps and volleying.	Jumping to the right, two beats per jump.
	16	Short jumps and volleying.	Jumping to the left, two beats per jump.
2	16	Jogging and volleying.	Jogging in place while volleying the ball back and forth to the center players. One step per beat.
3	16	Scissors jumps and volleying.	While volleying the ball back and forth to the center, do scissors jumps. Two beats per jump.
4	16	Jogging and volleying.	Same as in Part 2.

Repeat the routine until end of music.

INSTRUCTIONS:

This routine should be done using a circle formation. There can be 15-20 participants per circle with one to three participants in the center. The action of the different Parts is done while volleying the balls back and forth with center players. Center players also do the same movements as players in the circle. One to three beachballs is recommended per circle. This routine is designed for players of above average skills. Once routine starts, add clapping of hands to the beat of the music.

VOLLEYBALL

SKILLS: Bumping and Setting

MUSIC: "High on You" (Survivor)

EQUIPMENT: None

PARTS	BEATS	MOVEMENT	DESCRIPTION
1	16	Running.	In place.
	16	Shuffle bumping.	Two step side shuffle, one count step sideways, one count bump with forearms while raising shoulders, then repeat to other side using four counts. Go twice to each side.
2	16	Running.	In place.
	16	Sets.	Two steps forwards, dip elbows set with hands above head, 1/4 turn to left side and repeat using four counts to all four sides.
3	16	Running.	
	16	Shuffle bumping.	Same as in Part 1.
	16	Running.	
	16	Sets.	Same as in Part 2, except make 1/4 turns to right side.

Repeat the routine until end of music.

INSTRUCTIONS:

Imagery is recommended for participants of average or below skill levels. For the participants that have skill levels above average, volleyballs or beachballs maybe implemented.

VOLLEYBALL

SKILLS: Rotation, Bumping, and Setting

MUSIC: "Beat It" (Michael Jackson)

EQUIPMENT: None

PARTS	BEATS	MOVEMENT	DESCRIPTION
1	4	Jogging and arm circling.	Jog in place making large arm circles.
2	4	Running.	Rotate to your new place.
	16	Jumping jacks.	Four jumping jacks.
	4	Jogging and arm circling.	Jog in place making large arm circles.
3	4	Running.	Rotate to your new place.
	16	Bumping.	Eight bumps.
	4	Jogging and arm circling.	Jog in place making large arm circles.
4	4	Running.	Rotate to new place.
	16	Setting.	Eight sets.
	4	Jogging and arm circling.	Jog in place making large arm circles.
5	4	Running.	Rotate to new place.

Repeat the routine until end of music.

INSTRUCTIONS:

If participants are below average in skill level, imagery is recommended for the bumping and setting skills. For average and above, the
use of a beachball or volleyball would be appropriate. If a ball is
used, imagery would have to be used when the ball was not available
for a player to bump or set.

If a large group of participants is involved, it is possible to
organize the group in the following formations and rotate according to
the arrows.

```
XXXXXXXXXXXXXXXXXXXXXXXX        Net

→ O  →  O  →  O  →  O
                       ↓
↑ O  ←  O  ←  O  ←  O
  ↓
↑ O  →  O  →  O  →  O           Server
  ←      ←      ←      ↓
```

Player in serving position must run in double time to the front
position.

VOLLEYBALL

SKILLS: Volleying

MUSIC: "Rockin to Midnight"

EQUIPMENT: None

PARTS	BEATS	MOVEMENT	DESCRIPTION
1	4	Bumping.	Slide twice to right, lean down and bump.
	4	Bumping.	Slide twice to left, lean down and bump.
2	4	Jogging.	In place.
	4	Volleying.	Volley four times.
3	4	Jogging.	In place.
	4	Jumping.	Jump a square formation and a square lap to the beat of the music.

Repeat the routine until end of music.

INSTRUCTIONS:

Beachballs or volleyballs can be used with this routine, if the participants' skill levels are average or above. If the balls are not used, imagery is recommended. This routine is an excellent warm-up activity, unless the music is double taped and the routine repeated.

VOLLEYBALL

SKILLS: Bumping

MUSIC: "Elvira" (Oak Ridge Boys)

EQUIPMENT: One beachball or volleyball per circle.

PARTS	BEATS	MOVEMENT	DESCRIPTION
1	112	Sliding and bumping.	Student in circle slide counterclockwise. Person with beachball will bump it to someone across the circle who bumps it to someone else.
2	128	Sliding and bumping.	Circle changes to clockwise direction while continuing to bump.
	64	Sliding and bumping.	Circle changes to counter-clockwise direction.
	48	Sliding and bumping.	Circle changes to clockwise direction. Repeat if song would start after sixteen beats in this part.
	96	Sliding and bumping.	Circle changes to counter-clockwise direction.
	128	Sliding and bumping.	Circle changes to clockwise direction.
	64	Sliding and bumping.	Circle changes to counter-clockwise direction.
	32	Sliding and bumping.	Circle changes to clockwise direction.

INSTRUCTIONS:

It is necessary to double tape the music or repeat the song. The routine is designed for a repeat of the music. A circle formation is required.

VOLLEYBALL

SKILLS: Bumping and Jumping

MUSIC: "Working Day and Night"

EQUIPMENT: None

PARTS	BEATS	MOVEMENT	DESCRIPTION
1	16	Jumping jacks.	Two beats per jump. Do eight.
	8	Jumping.	To the right.
	8	Jumping.	To the left.
	16	Running.	In place.
2	4	Jogging.	Jog forward and bump on the fourth beat.
	4	Jogging.	Jog backward and bump on the fourth beat.

Repeat Part 2 three times.

| 3 | 16 | Running. | In place. |

Repeat the routine until end of music.

INSTRUCTIONS:

Imagery is recommended for the bumping skill execution. The routine is simple with good movement. The participant would have an opportunity to self analyze his/her bumping skills. Circle formation should be used.

VOLLEYBALL

SKILLS: Setting and Bumping

MUSIC: "Running in the Night" (Lionel Richie)

EQUIPMENT: One beachball or volleyball per two participants.

PARTS	BEATS	MOVEMENT	DESCRIPTION
1	16	Setting.	One half of the class with beachballs, set the ball for sixteen counts against the wall, the others jog in a large circle around the area.
2	8	Jogging and bumping.	Player with the ball jogs out to center of gym on the first six beats. Bump to a player without a ball or on the beats seven and eight.
3	8	Jogging.	Player now without ball start jogging for eight counts.

Repeat the routine until end of music.

INSTRUCTIONS:

A variety of organizational techniques may be used with this routine. Skill levels of the participants should be considered when organizing for this routine.

VOLLEYBALL

SKILLS: Bumping and Setting

MUSIC: "Lover Come Back To Me"

EQUIPMENT: None

PARTS	BEATS	MOVEMENT	DESCRIPTION
1	16	Bumping.	Straddle leg position, bump ball with hands, (shifting weight left to right) bump on second and fourth count.
2	16	Bumping.	Straddle leg position, further apart for a better stretch. Step together on the sixteenth count.
3	16	Setting and jumping.	Jump forward three counts, set on the fourth count. Set to each side forming a square, making quarter turns right.

Repeat the routine until end of music.

INSTRUCTIONS:

Imagery is recommended for this routine. If skill levels of participants are above average, then beachballs or volleyballs maybe used.

VOLLEYBALL

SKILLS: Serving, Bumping, Setting, Blocking and Spiking

MUSIC: "Y.M.C.A." (Men at Work)

EQUIPMENT: None

PARTS	BEATS	MOVEMENT	DESCRIPTION
1	24	Shake arms and bounce on heels.	Standing in place.
2	16	Underhand serving.	Left foot forward, slap palm in serving motion. Reverse, if left hand dominant. Make sixteen serves.
	16	Overhead serving.	Left arm overhead. Cock right arm and slap back of left hand in serving motion. Reverse, if left hand dominant.
	8	Jogging.	Standing in place.
3	32	Jogging, setting, blocking and spiking.	While jogging make one quarter turns to the right and complete a square formation. Make to set passes in between turns. Do a total of eight passes. Repeat, except block. Repeat, except spike. Repeat the square formation, except jog.
	32	Repeat Part 2.	
4	32	Bumping.	Get set, make four bumps forward, four to the right side, four forward, four to the left side. Do this two times. Sixteen beats per time.
	64	Repeat Part 3.	

Repeat the routine until end of music.

INSTRUCTIONS:

Imagery is recommended for this routine. Although no equipment is used, it is important for the participant to understand how to correctly execute the skills. If participants have advanced skill levels, it is possible to use volleyballs or beachballs.

VOLLEYBALL

SKILLS: Bumping and Serving

MUSIC: "How Will I Know"

EQUIPMENT: Volleyballs

PARTS	BEATS	MOVEMENT	DESCRIPTION
1	8	Jogging and serving.	Jogging in place, make two underhand or overhand serves. Serve should be made on fourth and eighth beat.
2	8	Jogging, serving and bumping.	Jogging in place, make overhand serve on fourth beat. Jump forward on first beat, toss ball up, bump and catch on next three beats.
	8	Jumping and bumping.	Jump forward of both feet, one jump per beat. Make four jumps, then toss ball up bump and catch on next four beats.
3	16	Jumping jacks.	Do eight, using two beats per jump. Lay ball on floor for this part.

Repeat the routine until music ends.

INSTRUCTIONS:

Beachballs or other light weight balls maybe used instead of volley-balls. If participants skill levels are below average, imagery is recommended.

VOLLEYBALL

SKILLS: Sliding and Bumping

MUSIC: "Rockin' at Midnight"

EQUIPMENT: Balloons or beachballs.

PARTS	BEATS	MOVEMENT	DESCRIPTION
1	16	Jumping jacks.	Holding balloon in front of body. Do eight.
2	4	Sliding and bumping.	Two sliding steps to the left and bump the balloon.
	4	Sliding bumping.	Two sliding steps to the right and bump the balloon.
3	8	Jogging.	Holding balloon in front of body jog eight steps in place.

Repeat the routine until end of music.

VOLLEYBALL

SKILLS: Volleying

MUSIC: "Physical" (Olivia Newton-John)

EQUIPMENT: Beachball or balloons.

PARTS	BEATS	MOVEMENT	DESCRIPTION
1	32	Volleying.	Volley a ball or balloon back and forth from one circle to the others.
2	32	Volleying.	Change directions and repeat the above.

Repeat the routine until end of music.

INSTRUCTIONS:

Form double circles. Outside circle jogs clockwise while inner circle jogs counter-clockwise. Circles change directions every thirty-two beats. Possible variations are: 1) Add a hand clap on every fourth beat, and 2) Add a balloon for volleying at the same time as the beachball. Double taping of the music is recommended.

VOLLEYBALL

SKILLS: Setting and Running

MUSIC: "California Girls" (David Lee Roth)

EQUIPMENT: Balloons

PARTS	BEATS	MOVEMENT	DESCRIPTION
1	8	Setting.	Make four sets using imagery. Two beats per set.
2	4	Running.	In proper rotating order, run to a new position and get ready to set.

Repeat the routine until end of music.

INSTRUCTIONS:

All players assume a place on court so they are in a game-like formation. If there are more players than what are on a normal volleyball team, adjustments can be made and extra positions added. Once the rotation system is learned, balloons can be added for setting. Double taping of the music is recommended for this routine to get extra exercise time.

VOLLEYBALL

SKILLS: Rotating, Serving, Bumping and Setting

MUSIC: "Star Wars"

EQUIPMENT: None

PARTS	BEATS	MOVEMENT	DESCRIPTION
1	8	Rotation and jogging.	Jog in place four beats and use four beats to rotate to a new position.
2	8	Setting, bumping and serving.	If on front row, do two sets, two beats per set. If on middle row, do two bumps, two beats per bump. If on back row, do two serves, two beats per serve. All rows do one jumping jack, using two beats.

Repeat the routine until end of music.

INSTRUCTIONS:

Imagery is recommended. If skill level of participants is above average, volleyballs or beachballs can be used.

VOLLEYBALL

SKILLS: Volleying and Setting

MUSIC: "All She Wants To Do Is Dance" (Don Henley)

EQUIPMENT: None

PARTS	BEATS	MOVEMENT	DESCRIPTION
1	4	Shuffle steps.	Feet moving up and down, standing in place.
	16	Shuffle steps and volleying.	Four counts, make a volley on the fourth beat moving side to side. Do this four times.
2	4	Shuffle steps.	Feet moving up and down, standing in place.
	16	Shuffle steps.	In a square with a half-turn, four count. First time, go right. Second time, go left. Then repeat. Make turn on each fourth count.
3	4	Shuffle steps.	Feet moving up and down, standing in place.
	16	Running and setting.	Four counts, run forward and set on the fourth count. Four count backward run, and repeat. Second time, go side to side and repeat. When setting, make sure knees and elbows are bent (always use correct imagery).

Repeat the routine until end of music.

INSTRUCTIONS:

Imagery is recommended for this routine. Balloons or light weight balls could be used depending on skill levels.

SELECTED BIBLIOGRAPHY

Johnson, P.B., Updyke, W.F., Schaefer, M., Stolberg, D.C. Sport Exercise and You. New York, NY: Holt, Rinehart, and Winston, 1975.

Morris, G.S. and Stiehl, J. Physical Education: From Intent to Action. Columbus, OH: Charles E. Merrill Publishing Company, 1985.

Scates, A.E. Winning Volleyball. 3rd ed. Dubuque, IA: Wm. C. Brown Publishers, 1988.

Scates, A.E. Winning Volleyball Drills. Dubuque, IA: Wm. C. Brown Publishers, 1988.

SKILLS USED IN TENNIS ROUTINES

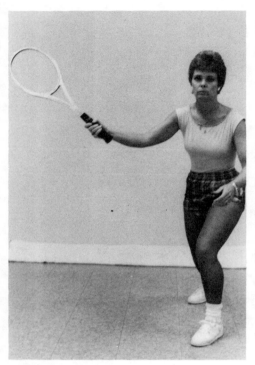

Forehand Stroke

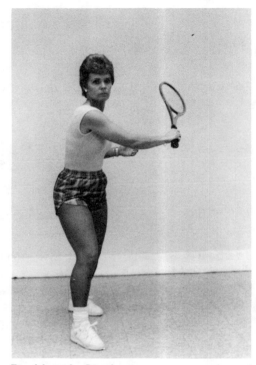

Backhand Stroke

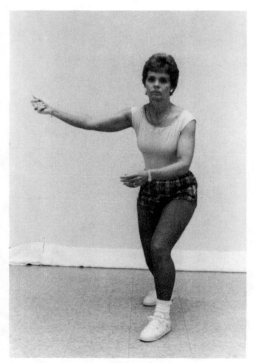

Forehand Stroke Without Racquet

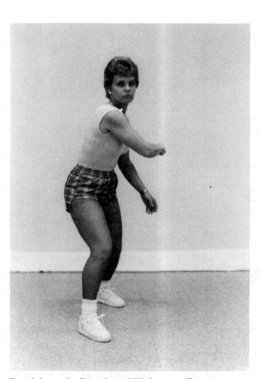

Backhand Stroke Without Racquet

CHAPTER 10

TENNIS

Tennis is a game that requires many different types of movements. When the body is in good condition and performance is with maximum efficiency, this game can be a very enjoyable experience. Without these qualities, the game can be very frustrating. In reality, it is no different than any other sport. Physical fitness is an important factor.

For many years, tennis in America was considered a "country club" type of sport. To many people that meant little or no opportunities were available to learn tennis skills let alone play the game. Until the 1960's, availability of courts and facilities were also a problem for the average American. During the late 1960's, tennis gained in popularity. More Americans were playing it and many began to see tennis as a game that could be played through the retirement years. More courts and facilities became available as cities, schools, and recreation agencies began to invest more money for these purposes. Technology also made drastic improvements in tennis equipment that helped individuals become more skilled. As people experienced success with this game, the interest increased. The visibility of tennis provided by television was probably another factor that generated interest in this sport. It seems apparent that the youth of today are interested in participating in the game of tennis. This would indicate that there will not be a demise in the ranks of tennis players for some time in the future.

One of the most significant advances for tennis has been the emphasis on it as a "lifetime" sport. There is a wide range of competitive situations available for all ages and skill levels. Whether tennis is played for serious competition or simply for fun and enjoyment, it is a very rewarding and enjoyable sport.

TENNIS AND FITNESS

Tennis is a game of starts and stops. As a result it is not classified as an aerobic exercise. This does not mean that general physical fitness and cardiovascular endurance is not important to successfully play tennis. Quite the contrary, having a good level of physical fitness can enhance the quality of skill execution in a game of tennis.

If an individual wishes to take the game of tennis seriously, a well rounded physical fitness program is needed. In order to execute tennis skills well an individual must demonstrate good power and strength, flexibility and cardiovascular endurance. As a result of these qualities, better performances can be expected.

Tennis Skills

Like many sports, tennis is a game that requires two different types of skills. First, an individual must develop those skills that are specific to the sport. Second, an individual must have good eye-hand coordination, eye-foot coordination, agility, and balance. The second group of skills are the fundamental motor skills required in most every sport. Since all of the skills that are specific to the sport must be executed on the move, it seems apparent that aerobic fitness will play a vital role in how well one learns and executes the skills.

The specific skills of tennis are: groundstrokes, serving, volleying, overheads, lobs, approach shots and drop shots. Since the game of tennis requires the use of a racquet other aspects of fitness are necessary. All of these skills require an individual to make a variety of movements. To execute these movements with proficiency, lower body conditioning is necessary.

Strength and Endurance

For the most part, tennis is a game that requires total body movement. Anytime a sport requires that an individual demonstrate a lot of movement, proper conditioning is very critical. Since tennis is a racquet sport, one must have enough strength to manipulate and control the racquet. Virtually every play in tennis requires leg movement, which means that leg strength is important. Total body strength is needed to experience successful play in tennis.

Tennis is known as a game with many short stops. These stops come after every point, when a ball is retrieved for play, and when court sides are changed after various games. To many people, this means that tennis is a sport that enables you to rest several times during a game. This is not an accurate assumption. Although there are starts and stops, most every point requires an individual to physically excel for a short period of time. There is a big difference in running several 100 yard sprints and jogging for a mile. Tennis is demanding of the cardiovascular system, especially when two players of equal ability are playing each other. Being aerobically fit is necessary, if one is to have the endurance required to play the sport. Once the action starts in this game, the movements are fast and demanding of an individual's physical ability.

TENNIS ROUTINES

The following sports aerobic routines were designed to help an individual develop or improve his/her basic tennis skills and at the same time develop a fitness level appropriate for the game. These routines can be easily changed or modified to better meet specific needs. If the routines are changed, it may require a change in the music used. The routines were developed around selected tennis skills. These skills are listed in Figure 10.1.

```
1.   Serving            4.   Volley
2.   Backhand Stroke    5.   Overheads
3.   Forehand Stroke    6.   Running
```

FIGURE 10.1   Basic tennis skills for which
the routines were developed.

The routines are few in number as compared to the numbers in other chapters. The reason for this was due to the difficulty of developing routines with a variety of movements. Tennis does not seem to a sport where variation in skills is obvious. This does mean that new tennis routines cannot be developed. The process of developing sport aerobic routines is outlined and discussed earlier in the text.

The routines are recommended for all ages. Once an individual starts to play tennis, all of the skills and movements in the routines are required to successfully play the game. The routines are designed to give an individual a workout that combines the practicing of tennis skills with an aerobic workout. These experiences should provide game like situations for the individual. Basically, the routines are a means to practice like you would play.

TENNIS

SKILLS: Forehand and Backhand Strokes

MUSIC: "Electric Avenue" (Eddy Grant)

EQUIPMENT: One tennis racquet per participant.

PARTS	BEATS	MOVEMENT	DESCRIPTION
1	16	Forehand strokes.	Execute four strokes. Use four beats per stroke.
	16	Backhand strokes.	Execute four strokes. Use four beats per stroke.
2	16	Sliding steps and forehand strokes.	Slide to the right (four beats) make a forehand stroke (four beats). Repeat.
	16	Sliding steps and backhand strokes.	Slide to the left (four beats) make a backhand stroke (four beats). Repeat.

Repeat all of Part 2.

PARTS	BEATS	MOVEMENT	DESCRIPTION
3	16	Jogging.	Hold racquet in ready position and jog in place for eight beats. Then jog to other side of net and get ready to repeat the routine.

Repeat the routine until end of music and alternating net sides.

INSTRUCTIONS:

Imagery may be used instead of tennis racquets. If imagery is used, it is important for the participant to develop a habit of analyzing his/her skills as the routine is performed. Without the racquet skill deviation may occur.

TENNIS

SKILLS: Net and Overhead Shots

MUSIC: "Electric Avenue" (Eddy Grant)

EQUIPMENT: One tennis racquet per participant.

PARTS	BEATS	MOVEMENT	DESCRIPTION
1	16	Net shots.	Ready position, jog in place four beats, then execute two net shots (two beats per shot).
	16	Overhead shots.	Same as above except use overhead shot.
2	16	Net shots.	Slide to the right (four beats) make two net shots (two beats per shot). Repeat to the left. Forehand shots to the right, backhand shots to the left.
	16	Overhead shots.	Run backwards for four beats, make two overhead shots (two beats per shot). Run forwards four beats and make two overhead shots (two beats per shot).

Repeat all of Part 2.

| 3 | 16 | Sprinting. | Holding racquet, sprint to the right (four beats), to the left (four beats), forwards (four beats) and backwards (four beats). |

Repeat the routine until end of music.

INSTRUCTIONS:

Imagery may be used instead of tennis racquets. This routine is recommended for those who have average to above average skill level. Emphasis should be on skill analysis, if imagery is used.

TENNIS

SKILLS: Serving

MUSIC: "Wanna Be Startin Something" (Michael Jackson)

EQUIPMENT: One tennis racquet per participant.

PARTS	BEATS	MOVEMENT	DESCRIPTION
1	8	Running.	In place with racquet.
2	16	Serving.	Run in place four beats, use four beats to execute a serve. Repeat this sequence.
3	8	Running.	In place with racquet double timing.
4	16	Serving.	Run in place four beats (double time), use four beats to execute a serve. Repeat this sequence.

Repeat the routine until end of music.

INSTRUCTIONS:

Imagery may also be used with this routine. Skill levels of the participants would be a determining factor. It would not be safe to do this routine in a small space, unless there were only a few participants.

TENNIS

SKILLS: Basic Movement

MUSIC: "Chain Reaction" (Diana Ross)

EQUIPMENT: One tennis racquet per participant.

PARTS	BEATS	MOVEMENT	DESCRIPTION
1	16	Running.	Holding the racquet in ready position, run in place for eight beats. On ninth beat sprint to a position on floor pretending to move in position for a shot. Use a total of eight beats.
	8	Jumping.	Lift racquet over head, and make four jumps. Two beats per jump.
2	16	Running.	Same as in the first segment of Part 1.
	8	Scissors jumps.	Holding the racquet in ready position do four scissors jumps. Two beats per jump.
3	16	Running.	Holding the racquet, run in different directions.

Repeat the routine until end of music.

INSTRUCTIONS:

Imagery is not recommended for this routine. It is best to use a racquet in order to receive the maximum effect of the exercise.

TENNIS

SKILLS: Forehand and Backhand Strokes

MUSIC: "Shakedown" (Bob Seger)

EQUIPMENT: One tennis racquet per participant.

PARTS	BEATS	MOVEMENT	DESCRIPTION
1	16	Forehand stroke and running.	Run in any direction for four beats, plant feet in ready position (two beats) and then make a forearm stroke (two beats). Repeat this sequence for another eight beats.
	16	Backhand stroke and running.	Use same sequence as above except execute a backhand stroke.
2	16	Net volleying.	Do eight net volleys using two beats per volley. Pretend you are four to six feet from the net.
	16	Overheads.	Do eight overheads at the net. Use two beats per overhead. Pretend you are six to eight feet from the net.
3	16	Running and lobs.	In a set position, assume ball has been hit over your head. Run back to lob the ball. Use four beats to run and four to make the shot. Repeat the sequence.
		Running.	Run forward for eight beats doing double time. Run backward for eight beats doing double time.

Repeat the routine until end of music.

SELECTED BIBLIOGRAPHY

Barra, R. G.   Basic Tennis: A Practical Guide for the Beginning
    Player. Minneapolis, NM: Burgess Publishing Company, 1984.

Collins, D. R., Hodges, P. B. and Haven, B. H.   Tennis: A Practical
    Learning Guide. Bloomington, IN: Tichenor Publishing, 1985.

Knight, B.   Practical Tennis: The Positive Way. Minneapolis, MN:
    Burgess Publishing Company, 1985.

Zebas, C. J. and Johnson, H. M.   Tennis: Back to the Basics.
    Dubuque, IA: Eddie Bowers Publishing Company, 1987.

SKILLS USED IN TRACK AND FIELD ROUTINES

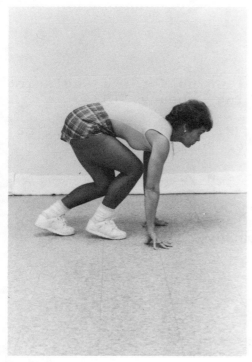

Sprinting

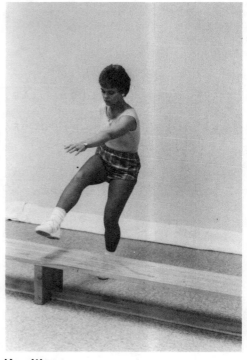

Hurdling

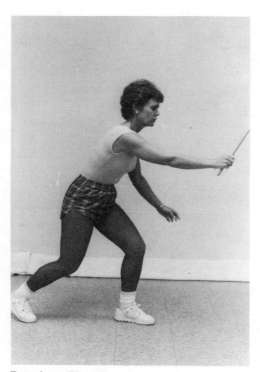

Passing The Baton

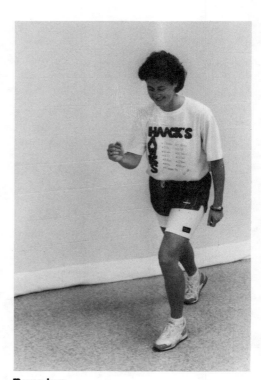

Running

CHAPTER 11

TRACK AND FIELD

It may seem strange to relate basic track and field skills to sport specific aerobic routines. On the other hand, why not? It is a sporting activity and requires a high level of physical fitness from those who participate in it. Track and field related activities appear to have increased in popularity during recent years. Upper elementary, junior high, and high school students have certainly shown more interest in this sport during the last 15 to 20 years. Older adults have shown more interest in this type of sport with increased numbers in walking and jogging programs.

Track and field activities are relatively easy to learn and easy to teach. For the most part the skills are also easy to learn. This is not to infer that the highly skilled track and field athlete has an easy time with performing the skills. The initial skills for a low level of competition seem to be somewhat easy for most people to develop. This may be another reason why the ranks of track and field participants seem to be increasing in numbers.

TRACK AND FIELD AND FITNESS

Track and field activities are a natural for developing physical fitness and aerobic fitness. Almost every track and field event or activity requires an individual to be in good physical condition. Since Americans are becoming conscious of their physical condition, more of them are seeking alternatives to traditional types of workout activities. These same individuals are beginning to realize that track and field activities have many different levels at which they can participate. More important is the fact that many of these activities are self paced. Simply, this means that an individual can learn the skills on a self-directed basis.

Today many people use track and field skills to develop and maintain their own fitness levels and state of well-being. For example, speed walking has become popular with many. Also, there are joggers, runners, sprinters and strength specialists in all age groups. Twenty years ago, most high school and college tracks were used only by the athletes. Today, these same tracks are used by many different people to promote aerobic fitness as well as physical fitness in general.

Track and Field Skills

All motor skills related to track and field activities require that an individual have good physical fitness for proper execution. Regardless of what type of physical fitness program in which one may be involved, the desire to improve is always evident. With improvement comes good skill development. Track and field activities are good for developing lower and upper body strength. The same activities can also provide positive results for the cardiovascular and respiratory systems.

The basic track and field skills that can aid in the development of physical and aerobic fitness are: running, sprinting, walking, jumping, hurdling and the shot put. Many young people today seem to have a growing interest in track and field skills and activities. It may be because many opportunities exist in this type of activity.

Strength and Endurance

To properly and successfully execute the skills previously discussed, strength and endurance are necessary qualities. If an individual has a low level of total body strength and poor endurance, consistent and regular participation in track and field activities may improve these qualities. In fact for the individual who is looking for a workout alternative, track and field activities must be viewed in this manner.

It is important to consider track and field activities like any other sport. All sports can be used as tools to improve personal fitness and well being. For one to improve and maintain strength and endurance by using track and field activities, participation must be regular and consistent. The more these individual qualities improve, the greater the enjoyment.

TRACK AND FIELD ROUTINES

The sport aerobic routines in this chapter were designed for an individual to improve his/her skills in track and field activities as well as in the area of aerobic fitness. These routines can be easily modified or changed to meet specific needs. If a change is made, it may be necessary to change the music. A variety of different music may also be used for each routine. The routines were developed around selected track and field skills. These skills are listed in Figure 11.1

```
1.  Jumping        4.  Shot Putting
2.  Running        5.  Sprinting
3.  Hurdling       6.  Discuss Throwing
```

Figure 11.1 Basic track and field skills for
            which the routines were developed.

There are less of these routines than for some of the other sports. It is difficult to develop routines for this particular sport that show variation. In fact, it is best to work with one basic routine and expand or add parts as the participants learn it. For developing new routines, one should follow the process outlined in an earlier chapter of this text.

TRACK AND FIELD

<u>SKILLS</u>: Jumping, Shot Putting, and Hurdling

<u>MUSIC</u>:   Old Time Rock'n Roll (Bob Seger)

<u>EQUIPMENT</u>: None

PARTS	BEATS	MOVEMENT	DESCRIPTION
1	16	Hurdling.	Run clockwise, on seventh and eighth beats do a hurdle jump. Repeat the sequence, except jump on beats fifteen and sixteen.
	16	Hurdling.	Same as above, except run counterclockwise.
2	4	Running.	Running in place, raising knees high. Take four steps, one step per beat.
	4	Shot putting.	Pivot on the first two beats and then throw the shot on beats three and four.

Repeat Part 2.

PARTS	BEATS	MOVEMENT	DESCRIPTION
3	8	Running/sprinting and jumping.	Run or sprint for four beats, make a long jump on beats five and six. Use beats seven and eight to recover and get ready to repeat.
	8	Running/sprinting and jumping.	Same as above.

Repeat the routine until music ends.

<u>INSTRUCTIONS</u>:

Imagery is recommended for the hurdling and shot putting. It would be possible to do this routine with hurdles placed at random positions on the floor. Small soft textured balls could also be used as the shots.

TRACK AND FIELD

SKILLS: Discuss Throwing

MUSIC: "Holiday Hotel" (Loggins and Messina)

EQUIPMENT: None

PARTS	BEATS	MOVEMENT	DESCRIPTION
1	8	Throwing.	Make three swings and on the third release discus and follow through with body. Two beats per swing and throw discus on beats seven and eight.
2	16	Running.	Run through space for fourteen beats, use the last two beats to get set for throwing.

Repeat the routine until end of music.

INSTRUCTIONS:

Imagery is recommended when throwing the discus. It is possible to use a frisbee as a discus. One frisbee would be needed per participant. Skill level of the participants should be considered as to whether or not any type of equipment is used with the routine.

TRACK AND FIELD

SKILLS: Sprinting and Baton Passing

MUSIC: "Chain Reaction" (Diana Ross)

EQUIPMENT: Batons

PARTS	BEATS	MOVEMENT	DESCRIPTION
1	16	Jogging.	All jog in place with last one in line holding the baton.
	8	Passing baton.	During this eight beats the pass is made from the last in line to the next. All continue to run.
2	16	Sprinting.	All in the line sprint.
	8	Passing the baton.	Same as in Part 1.
3	16	Repeat Part 1.	Same as in Part 1.
	8	Repeat second phase of Part 2.	
4	16	Repeat Part 2.	Same as in Part 2.
	8	Repeat second phase of Part 2.	

Repeat the routine until music ends.

INSTRUCTIONS:

It is recommended that this routine be performed by organizing the participants into lines of six to eight. The distance between each individual can be determined by the instructor.

TRACK AND FIELD

SKILLS: Triple, Long and Scissor Jumping

MUSIC: "Junku" (Herbie Hancock)
Official Music of the XXIIIrd Olympiad -- Los Angeles, 1984

EQUIPMENT: Mats, high jump bars and standards

PARTS	BEATS	MOVEMENT	DESCRIPTION
1	16	Sprinting.	Line to prepare for a jump. Start in scattered formation and sprint to line up at the mat.
2	8	Triple jumping.	Use four beats on the approach, four beats to jump.
	16	Running.	Toward a high jump station. Should be in line on sixteenth beat.
3	8	Scissor jumping.	Over a bar, try various heights each time. Use four beats on the approach, four beats on the jump.
	16	Sprinting.	Toward a mat to line up for the long jump.
4	8	Long jumping.	Land on a mat only. Use four beats for the approach, four beats for the jump.
	16	Running.	Toward a high jump station.

Repeat the routine until end of music.

INSTRUCTIONS:

It is important for the participants to jog in place while in line to jump. This will help keep constant movement. Participants should be allowed to jump different heights as the routine is repeated. The instructor can change the height of the bar once a group has finished jumping. It is possible to split a large group into three groups, with one group at each station. The only difference would be the sequence of jumps.

TRACK AND FIELD

SKILLS: Starting Position for Dashes

MUSIC: "Dancing on the Ceiling" (Lionel Ritchie)

EQUIPMENT: One jump rope per participant

PARTS	BEATS	MOVEMENT	DESCRIPTION
1	8	Sprinting.	Begin in starting position and sprint to the rope.
	8	Jumping.	Forward and backward over the rope. One beat per jump.
2	4	Pick-up rope.	Get ready to jump.
	24	Rope jumping.	Jump rope using one beat per jump. Any jumping style may be used.
	8	Sprinting.	Use two beats to drop rope and get in starting position. Sprint for six beats.
3	8	Starter position hops.	Alternate legs with hands on floor.
4	8	Sprinting.	Forward to a rope.
4	4	Pick up rope.	Get set.
	16	Rope jumping.	Alternating feet and lifting knees high. One beat per jump.
	8	Sprinting.	Drop rope and sprint for six beats and get in starting position on beats seven and eight.

Repeat the routine until end of music.

SELECTED BIBLIOGRAPHY

Morris, G.S. and Stiehl, J. Physical Education: From Intent to Action. Columbus, OH: Charles E. Merrill Publishing Company, 1985.

Powell, J.R. Track and Field Fundamentals for Teacher and Coach, (3rd ed.). Champaign, ILL: Stipes Publishing Company, 1971.

Sorani, R. Circuit Training. Dubuque, IA: Wm. C. Brown Company, 1966.

CHAPTER **12**

EVALUATION AND ASSESSMENT

Adding exercise or changing exercise habits to everyday living is not always an easy thing to do. The addition of sport aerobic routines to an existing exercise program may be difficult at first because of the nature of the activity. It will also be difficult, at first, for an individual to start an exercise program using sport aerobic routines. Regardless of the inconvenience, sport aerobic activities will help you look and feel better. Sport aerobic routines and activities are no different than any other form of exercise. Progression is the "key" to a safe workout. Before attempting sport aerobic routines, you should know your current level of fitness. An evaluation of your fitness can help determine your exercise needs and keep you within safe limitations for a good workout.

It is important to assess the sport aerobic routines in relation to the participant's sport specific skills. Basic skills are necessary for one to have in order to receive an aerobic workout with these routines. The more that an individual is skilled in a particular sport, the greater the intensity of the workout.

ASSESSING PHYSICAL FITNESS FOR AEROBIC EXERCISE

Before attempting to participate in any exercise program or continuing in one, it is important for the individual to know his/her current level of fitness. Measuring fitness is the only way to determine individual needs and provide a safe avenue for exercising on a regular basis. This is also a good means for establishing personal goals. Before starting an exercise program, a thorough medical examination by a physician is recommended.

Aerobic Capacity

Before participating in sport aerobic routines, it is necessary for one to assess his/her aerobic capacity. This simply has to do with measuring the heart's response to increasing amounts of exercise by measuring one's ability to use oxygen. Aerobic exercise conditions the body's oxygen transport system to process the use of oxygen more efficiently. This transportation system is the heart, lungs, blood, and blood vessels. Since aerobic capacity depends upon the efficiency of this system, it becomes a good measure of overall physical fitness.

Measuring Aerobic Capacity

The measurement of aerobic capacity is important before getting into aerobic exercise, simply for the safety of the individual. By measuring aerobic capacity and assessing physical fitness, progression in exercise can better be determined. The key is to start exercising or continue exercising within the limitations of one's physical fitness level.

Measurement of aerobic capacity can be done in one of two different ways. First, it can be measured in a laboratory physical fitness test. Generally, in this setting, a sub-maximal or maximal test is administered. The laboratory director or test administrator usually determine which test is needed for the individual. Second, aerobic capacity can be measured by various field tests. This type of test may be administered individually, with a small group, or with a large group. Field tests are useful, especially if access to a laboratory and an exercise physiologist is unavailable.

Aerobic exercise should be a lifetime habit, therefore regular assessment of physical fitness is necessary to order to follow a progressive workout program. The assessment is also important for maintaining a good level of physical fitness. The following field tests are recommended for measuring aerobic capacity and assessing physical fitness.

1.   Cooper's 12-Minute Run/Walk Test.
2.   Cooper's 1.5 Mile Run/Walk Test.
3.   Harvard Step Test.
4.   One Minute Step Test.
5.   One Mile Run/Walk Test (Recommended for elementary
      and high school students).

Charts and tables with norms for all of these tests are available in numerous books, journals and other publications. If the One Mile Run/Walk Test is used for children and high school students, the American Alliance for Health, Physical Education, Recreation and Dance norms are recommended. The proper protocol for each test should be followed in order to get good feedback. It is necessary to use only one of these tests, unless for some reason the results do not appear to be correct. Should this be the case, it would then be necessary to repeat the test or select another test.

Using Test Results

Once the assessment has been made and the results obtained, it is important for the individual to understand this information. Regardless of the type of test (laboratory or field) used, the results would have to be at least good or better. With results of good or better, one should be physically fit enough to participate in sport aerobics with continuous movement over a period of time. If the results were below good, one should assume that the physical fitness level is low and start with an aerobics program involving less movement and a shorter period of exercise time.

A good guide to follow, after the test results have been obtained, is the "progressive overload principle." Sport specific aerobic routines can condition and strengthen the heart through this principle. These routines "overload" the heart by causing it to beat faster during a vigorous exercise workout. As a result, this makes for a temporary high demand on the cardiorespiratory system. As the physical fitness level improves, the intensity of the activity and the amount of exercise time may increase. If this principle is followed, an individual can safely improve his/her overall physical fitness and cardiovascular endurance.

Test measurements of aerobic capacity and cardiovascular endurance reflect the condition of the heart, blood vessels and lungs as well as the general condition of the muscles. For these reasons, participation in sport aerobics can improve one's cardiorespiratory system and general muscle condition during the same activity.

EVALUATION OF THE ROUTINES

The term "sport specific aerobic routines" implies physical fitness by working to strengthen the cardiorespiratory system. For this reason, it is important to evaluate each routine to determine if the required movement is aerobic in nature. This is not to say that if the movement is something other than aerobic, the routine should be discarded. Any routine that requires movement will be helpful toward improving an individual's overall physical condition, although it may not be truly aerobic.

Sport aerobic routines can be an exciting and challenging fitness activity. It combines basic motor skills with sport specific skills in a rhythmical setting. All movement is rhythmical, therefore it seems only logical that sport skills be practiced with music or some type of rhythmical medium. There are several criteria for assessing sport aerobic routines. It is well to remember that the evaluation is of the "movement in the routine" and not to determine the results after one has participated in it. Basically the evaluation should determine whether or not the routine is aerobic and sport specific. The following criteria are recommended to be used for evaluating existing routines or newly developed ones.

1. <u>Time</u> — Each routine should provide a workout of 15-20 minutes in length. For many of the routines in this book, it was recommended to <u>double</u> tape the music. It is also possible to use two different pieces of music to get the desired time.

2. <u>Continuous Movement</u> — All movements in the routine should be sequenced in such a way that it is easy for an individual to maintain nonstop movement for 15-20 minutes.

3. <u>Sport Specific Skills</u> — These skills should be easily adaptable to aerobic type movement.

4. <u>Music</u> — The music selected for a routine should have a steady, easy to follow beat. The beat should be conducive to aerobic movements.

5. Equipment - The routine should not require more equipment than what is available. If each participant is to have a ball, then enough balls must be available.

6. Skill Level - This is an important factor for sport specific aerobic routines. The skill level of the participants must be equal to the level of skills required in the routine.

7. Participants - Sport aerobic routines are for various age levels. There are differences in the types of routines that can be used for 12-13 year olds as compared to 40-45 year olds. When considering participants, other criteria, such as skill level, must be used as a determining factor.

These criteria are intended to serve as helpful guidelines for evaluating new routines and in the selection of existing routines for a particular individual or group. Most important is to use routines for the desired sport. When individuals have an interest in a particular sport, it is certainly going to make a difference in whether or not they accept sport specific aerobics as a form of exercise.

SUMMARY

Evaluation and assessment of physical fitness levels in individuals is very important prior to participating in sport aerobic routines. It is equally important to evaluate or assess the level of aerobic movement required in a routine. If the movements in a routine are not aerobic in nature, overall cardiovascular endurance may not be greatly affected.

In the assessment of physical fitness, the aerobic capacity of the individual must be the deciding factor as to the type and amount of exercise one can do. An appropriate test should be used to evaluate this variable. Ideally, a sub-maximal or maximal test in a laboratory should be used. If this type of test is not available, there are several recommended field tests.

Once the evaluation of the individual's physical fitness is complete, the results must be used accordingly. The progressive overload principle should be followed as one plans or continues an aerobic workout program. Properly using test results can help an individual safely participate in sport specific aerobic routines.

Finally, it is important to evaluate the routines to determine whether or not desired outcomes can be attained. The movements in each routine are specific to a specific sport. It is critical that the routine allow for the practicing of selected sport skills in a game like manner. This practice should be done aerobically. Each sport aerobic routine should also be fun to do, challenging and a good workout.

SELECTED BIBLIOGRAPHY

Garrison, L. and Read, A. Fitness for Every Body. Palo Alto, CA: Mayfield Publishing Company, 1980.

Mazzeo, K. and Kisselle, J. Aerobic Dance. (Alt. ed). Englewood, CO: Morton Publishing Company, 1984.

McGlynn, G. Dynamics of Fitness. Dubuque, IA: Wm. C. Brown Publishers, 1987.

Stokes, R., Moore, A.C., Moore, C. and Williams, C. Fitness: The New Wave. Winston-Salem, NC: Hunter Textbooks, Inc., 1981.

Thomas, T.R. Muscular Training Through Resistance Training. Dubuque, IA: Eddie Bowers Publishing Company, 1986.